Macular Edema: The Current Recommendations for Clinical Practice

Macular Edema: The Current Recommendations for Clinical Practice

Editor

Gawecki Maciej

MDPI • Basel • Beijing • Wuhan • Barcelona • Belgrade • Manchester • Tokyo • Cluj • Tianjin

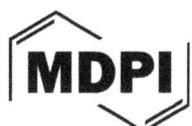

Editor
Gawecki Maciej
Ophthalmology
Dobry Wzrok Centrum
Okulistyczne
Gdansk
Poland

Editorial Office
MDPI
St. Alban-Anlage 66
4052 Basel, Switzerland

This is a reprint of articles from the Special Issue published online in the open access journal *Journal of Clinical Medicine* (ISSN 2077-0383) (available at: www.mdpi.com/journal/jcm/special_issues/Macular_Edema).

For citation purposes, cite each article independently as indicated on the article page online and as indicated below:

LastName, A.A.; LastName, B.B.; LastName, C.C. Article Title. *Journal Name* **Year**, *Volume Number*, Page Range.

ISBN 978-3-0365-3257-8 (Hbk)
ISBN 978-3-0365-3256-1 (PDF)

© 2022 by the authors. Articles in this book are Open Access and distributed under the Creative Commons Attribution (CC BY) license, which allows users to download, copy and build upon published articles, as long as the author and publisher are properly credited, which ensures maximum dissemination and a wider impact of our publications.

The book as a whole is distributed by MDPI under the terms and conditions of the Creative Commons license CC BY-NC-ND.

Contents

About the Editor vii

Preface to "Macular Edema: The Current Recommendations for Clinical Practice" ix

Maciej Gawecki
Subthreshold Diode Micropulse Laser Combined with Intravitreal Therapy for Macular Edema—A Systematized Review and Critical Approach
Reprinted from: *J. Clin. Med.* 2021, *10*, 1394, doi:10.3390/jcm10071394 1

Andrzej Grzybowski, Agne Markeviciute and Reda Zemaitiene
Treatment of Macular Edema in Vascular Retinal Diseases: A 2021 Update
Reprinted from: *J. Clin. Med.* 2021, *10*, 5300, doi:10.3390/jcm10225300 9

Slawomir Jan Teper
Update on the Management of Uveitic Macular Edema
Reprinted from: *J. Clin. Med.* 2021, *10*, 4133, doi:10.3390/jcm10184133 25

Michał Orski and Maciej Gawecki
Current Management Options in Irvine–Gass Syndrome: A Systemized Review
Reprinted from: *J. Clin. Med.* 2021, *10*, 4375, doi:10.3390/jcm10194375 39

Izabella Karska-Basta, Weronika Pociej-Marciak, Michał Chrzaszcz, Agnieszka Kubicka-Trzaska, Magdalena Debicka-Kumela and Maciej Gawecki et al.
Imbalance in the Levels of Angiogenic Factors in Patients with Acute and Chronic Central Serous Chorioretinopathy
Reprinted from: *J. Clin. Med.* 2021, *10*, 1087, doi:10.3390/jcm10051087 53

Maciej Gawecki
Idiopathic Peripheral Retinal Telangiectasia in Adults: A Case Series and Literature Review
Reprinted from: *J. Clin. Med.* 2021, *10*, 1767, doi:10.3390/jcm10081767 67

Ewa Kosior-Jarecka, Dominika Wróbel-Dudzińska, Anna Święch and Tomasz Żarnowski
Bleb Compressive Sutures in the Management of Hypotony Maculopathy after Glaucoma Surgery
Reprinted from: *J. Clin. Med.* 2021, *10*, 2223, doi:10.3390/jcm10112223 83

Mateusz Winiarczyk, Dagmara Winiarczyk, Katarzyna Michalak, Kai Kaarniranta, Łukasz Adaszek and Stanisław Winiarczyk et al.
Dysregulated Tear Film Proteins in Macular Edema Due to the Neovascular Age-Related Macular Degeneration Are Involved in the Regulation of Protein Clearance, Inflammation, and Neovascularization
Reprinted from: *J. Clin. Med.* 2021, *10*, 3060, doi:10.3390/jcm10143060 95

Chiara Altana, Matthew Gavino Donadu, Stefano Dore, Giacomo Boscia, Gabriella Carmelita and Stefania Zanetti et al.
Clinical Outcome and Drug Expenses of Intravitreal Therapy for Diabetic Macular Edema: A Retrospective Study in Sardinia, Italy
Reprinted from: *J. Clin. Med.* 2021, *10*, 5342, doi:10.3390/jcm10225342 109

About the Editor

Gawecki Maciej

Maciej Gawecki, Md PhD is a graduate of Medical University in Gdansk, Poland. His PhD covers the subject of amblyopia, however his interests since then shifted towards medical retina, including modern diagnostics and treatment, especially application of non-damaging forms of laser. At present, Dr Gawecki heads his own ophthalmological clinic: Dobry Wzrok in Gdansk and coordinates Department of Ophthalmology of Specialist Hospital in Chojnice, Poland. He also takes the position of regional consultant for pomorskie province in Poland in the field of ophthalmology.

Preface to "Macular Edema: The Current Recommendations for Clinical Practice"

Dear readers,

We invite you to read a few articles that cover the broad subject of macular edema. Macular edema is a common clinical entity that has variable etiopathogenic background. Advances in ophthalmological technology, especially the advent of OCT –angiography, have made diagnostics of that syndrome more profound and shed a different light into its classifications and therapeutic approaches. On the other hand, introduction of intravitreal therapies to ophthalmological practice has revolutionized treatment of macular edema and gave a different perspective for the use of classical laser photocoagulation in such cases. It also made research redirect towards non-damaging retinal therapies such as subthreshold laser treatment applied in pulsed mode. No matter how we appreciate advances in the diagnostics and treatment of macular edema, there are still many issues that remain a medical mystery. That situation, sometimes, has a consequence in the lack of strong therapeutic recommendations supported by relevant research. This book is a presentation of discussions and experience of authors whose efforts aim towards creating precise recommendations for the treatment of macular edema in different ophthalmological diseases, including combination of intravitreal injections with other forms of treatment.

Gawecki Maciej
Editor

Review

Subthreshold Diode Micropulse Laser Combined with Intravitreal Therapy for Macular Edema—A Systematized Review and Critical Approach

Maciej Gawęcki

Dobry Wzrok Ophthalmological Clinic, Kliniczna 1B/2, 80-402 Gdańsk, Poland; gawecki@use.pl; Tel.: +48-501-788-654

Abstract: Objective: intravitreal therapy for macular edema (ME) is a common clinical approach to treating most retinal vascular diseases; however, it generates high costs and requires multiple follow-up visits. Combining intravitreal anti–vascular endothelial growth factor (VEGF) or steroid therapy with subthreshold diode micropulse laser (SDM) application could potentially reduce the burden of numerous intravitreal injections. This review sought to explore whether this combination treatment is effective in the course of ME secondary to retinal vascular disease, and in particular, determine whether it is comparable or superior to intravitreal therapy alone. Materials and methods: the following terms and Boolean operators were used to search the PubMed literature database: subthreshold micropulse laser, subthreshold diode micropulse OR micropulse laser treatment AND anti-VEGF, anti-VEGF treatment, intravitreal steroids, OR combined therapy.This analysis included all studies discussing the combination of SDM and intravitreal anti-VEGF or steroid treatment. Results: the search revealed nine studies that met the inclusion criteria, including five comparing combined treatment and anti-VEGF treatment alone, four covering diabetic ME, and one covering ME secondary to branch retinal vein occlusion. All of these five studies suggested that combination therapy results in fewer intravitreal injections than anti-VEGF monotherapy with non-inferior functional and morphological outcomes. The remaining four studies report functional and morphological improvements after combined treatment; however, SDM alone was never superior to intravitreal-alone or combined treatment. There were substantial differences in treatment protocols and inclusion criteria between the studies. Conclusions: the available material was too scarce to provide a reliable assessment of the effects of combined therapy and its relation to intravitreal monotherapy in the treatment of ME secondary to retinal vascular disease. One assumption of note is that it is possible that SDM plus anti-VEGF might require fewer intravitreal injections than anti-VEGF monotherapy with equally good functional and morphological results. However, further randomized research is required to confirm this thesis.

Keywords: combined treatment; subthreshold diode micropulse; anti-VEGF treatment; diabetic macular edema; retinal vein occlusion

1. Introduction

Subthreshold diode micropulse laser (SDM) therapy has been used extensively to treat retinal disorders in recent years [1,2]. The efficacy of SDM in the treatment of central serous chorioretinopathy (CSCR) has been proven in numerous studies and accepted as a routine form of treatment by many ophthalmologists in the context of this specific disease [3–5].

However, in other retinal disorders, especially vascular ones, current recommendations emphasize the application of intravitreal therapies. In this context, the use of SDM in these diseases remains an area to be explored. Functional improvements after SDM alone in the treatment of macular edema (ME) or diabetic ME (DME) secondary to retinal vein occlusion (RVO), can generally be described as moderate and not superior to gains achieved after intravitreal therapies [6]. On the other hand, real-world studies suggest that the actual visual gains achieved after intravitreal therapy are usually smaller than those reported in the randomized clinical trials that were the basis for the drug's approval [7,8]. Additionally, the dense schedule of intravitreal therapy places a substantial burden on the patients, contrary to when undergoing laser treatment, which is performed less frequently. This fact was proved by reviewing five years of results of the Protocol S study by the Diabetic Retinopathy Clinical Research Network, which compared the efficacy of pan-retinal photocoagulation versus intravitreal ranibizumab for proliferative diabetic retinopathy [9]. As much as one-third of patients did not complete the trial, which often resulted in the serious progression of diabetic retinopathy. However, deterioration was much more frequent in noncompliant patients from the ranibizumab group than in those from the laser group. In light of this knowledge, the question of SDM application in retinal vascular diseases could be asked in a different way: is SDM capable of reducing the number of necessary intravitreal injections needed to maintain vision? The goal of this review was to analyze the effects of the combination of SDM and intravitreal injections in DME and ME secondary to RVO based on the available literature. In particular, the present review seeks to find premises in which to use SDM as a supportive therapy that would reduce the number of necessary intravitreal injections.

2. Materials and Methods

The following terms and Boolean operators together were used to search the PubMed literature database: subthreshold micropulse laser, subthreshold diode micropulse OR micropulse laser treatment AND anti-VEGF, anti-VEGF treatment, intravitreal steroids, OR combined therapy. The present analysis included all available studies that involved the combination of SDM and intravitreal anti-vascular endothelial growth factor (VEGF) or steroid treatment within the years: 2000–2021 in the PubMed database. Both SDM and anti-VEGF treatment were not available before 2000.

3. Results

The search revealed nine studies altogether that involved combined SDM with intravitreal treatment in ME, with the oldest one indexed in 2008. Five of these compared the results of combination treatment to those of intravitreal therapy alone. A description of these trials is presented in Table 1.

Table 1. Studies that compared combined SDM and anti-VEGF/intravitreal steroid therapy and intravitreal treatment alone in the management of retinal diseases.

Author/Year of Publication	Material	Study Design	Results
DME			
Thinda et al. 2014 [10]	anti-VEGF + SDM (n = 10 eyes); anti-VEGF (n = 10 eyes)	Retrospective; evaluation of the number of injections and improvements in BCVA and CRT; follow-up of six to 18 months with a median of 12 months	Mean number of injections per month: 0.27 in the combined group and 0.67 in anti-VEGF group (difference was statistically significant); significant improvements in BCVA and final CRT similar in both groups.
Moisseiev et al. 2018 [11]	IVR + SDM (n = 19 eyes); IVR (n = 19 eyes)	Retrospective; comparison of BCVA and number of injections in both groups at 12 months and at the end of the follow-up; most patients in the SDM group had CRT < 400 µm; no more than three IVRs before SDM application.	Significant BCVA improvement similar in both groups; number of required injections was significantly fewer in the combined group than in the monotherapy group: 1.7 ± 2.3 vs. 5.6 ± 2.1 at 12 months and 2.6 ± 3.3 vs. 9.3 ± 5.1 at the end of follow-up.

Table 1. Cont.

Author/Year of Publication	Material	Study Design	Results
Khattab et al. 2019 [12]	DME IVA (n = 27 eyes); SDM + IVA (n = 27 eyes)	Prospective, randomized; impact of adjuvant SDM therapy as compared with aflibercept treatment alone on the number of injections; evaluation of the number of injections, BCVA, and CS at 18 months; SDM applied within one week after the loading phase of injections.	Number of injections in the aflibercept group was 7.3 vs. 4.1 in the combined group (difference significant); BCVA improved significantly by a similar amount in both groups; CS improved significantly in both groups by a similar degree.
Kanar et al. 2020 [13]	DME IVA (n = 28 eyes); IVA + SDM (n = 28 eyes)	Prospective RCT; comparison of BCVA, CRT, and number of injections required in both groups at 12 months; SDM applied after at least three loading doses of IVA and until CRT decreased below 450 μm.	IVA group experienced significant BCVA improvement from 0.38 ± 0.1 logMAR to 0.20 ± 0.1 logMAR and CRT reduction from 451.28 ± 44.85 μm to 328.8 ± 49.69 μm, while the combined group experienced significant BCVA improvement from 0.40 ± 0.09 logMAR to 0.17 ± 0.06 logMAR and CRT reduction from 466.07 ± 71.79 μm to 312.0 ± 39.29 μm—thus, no statistically significant differences in BCVA and CRT changes existed between the groups; the number of injections in the combined group was significantly smaller than in the monotherapy group at 3.21 ± 0.41 vs. 5.39 ± 1.54.
	BRVO		
Terashima et al. 2019 [14]	ME secondary to BRVO IVR group (n = 24 eyes); IVR + SDM group (n = 22 eyes)	Retrospective; evaluation of BCVA, CRT, and number of injections in both groups at six months; SDM performed one month after initial IVR; IVR applied in PRN fashion after the first initial injection in both groups.	BCVA and CRT improved significantly in both groups without significant differences; combined group required statistically fewer injections than the IVR monotherapy group (1.9 ± 0.8 vs. 2.3 ± 0.9) by three months.

SDM, subthreshold diode micropulsation; IVR, intravitreal ranibizumab; IVA, intravitreal aflibercept; IVT, intravitreal triamcinolone; BCVA, best-corrected visual acuity; CRT, central retinal thickness; ME, macular edema; BRVO, branch retinal vein occlusion; DME, diabetic macular edema; CS, contrast sensitivity; RCT, randomized clinical trial; PRN, pro re nata; VEGF, vascular endothelial growth factor.

The studies compared in Table 1 consist of four studies covering DME [10–13] and one study concerning ME secondary to branch retinal vein occlusion (BRVO) [14]. Among those studies, there were two randomized clinical trials on DME by Khattab et al. [12] and Kanar et al. [13], respectively. The results of combined anti-VEGF plus SDM treatment were compared with the outcomes of anti-VEGF. These five studies reported similar best-corrected visual acuity (VA) (BCVA) and retinal morphology improvements in both groups, with significantly fewer injections required in the combined therapy cohort. Moreover, in all of these studies, SDM was performed after the loading phase of the intravitreal injection; however, the number of loading injections varied across the studies. Subsequent treatment with anti-VEGF medications was conducted in a pro re nata fashion.

Each of the remaining four studies had a unique design and they did not include intravitreal therapy alone as a reference. Nevertheless, they were analyzed because they documented the results of combined therapy. Two trials compared the outcome of combination treatment versus SDM alone [15,16], and two studies presented the effects of combination treatment in specific cases of ME [17,18]. A description of these four studies is provided in Table 2.

Table 2. Studies that assessed the combination of SDM and intravitreal treatment without results for intravitreal therapy alone.

Author/Year of Publication	Material	Study Design	Results
		BRVO	
Parodi et al. 2008 [15]	ME secondary to BRVO SDM (n = 13 eyes) (810 nm) SDM + IVT (n = 11 eyes)	Prospective RCT; comparison of BCVA between the groups at 12 months.	Gain of at least 10 ETDRS letters in 91% of eyes in the SDM + IVT group and in 62% of eyes in the SDM-alone group; mean number of lines gained: 3.4 in the SDM + IVT group and 1.3 in the SDM-alone groups (the difference between the groups was significant).
		DME	
Luttrull et al. 2012 [16]	DME SDM (n = 38 eyes); SDM + anti-VEGF or IVT (n = 24 eyes); SDM-alone group had significantly smaller CRT at baseline	Retrospective; evaluation of BCVA and CRT after treatment (median follow up 12 months); SDM followed intravitreal therapy.	Significant reduction in CRT in 71% of the SDM-alone group and 89.5% of the combination group (with no statistical difference between the groups); BCVA stable in both groups, but without significant improvement.
Elhamid 2017 [17]	DME resistant to anti-VEGF therapy Ozurdex* plus SDM (n = 20 eyes)	Case series; evaluation of BCVA and CRT at 12 months; SDM performed at one month after injection of Ozurdex; possible reinjection at six months.	BCVA was significantly improved from 0.45 $\pm$ 0.14 to 0.59 $\pm$ 0.14 Snellen, while CRT was significantly reduced from 420.7 $\pm$ 38.74 µm to 285.2 $\pm$ 14.99 µm; reinjection was necessary in eight eyes; cataract was present in six of 14 phakic eyes.
Inagaki et al. 2019 [18]	DME SDM + anti-VEGF (n = 34 eyes, including 27 IVR and 7 IVA)	Retrospective; evaluation of BCVA, CRT, and the number of injections at 12 months; loading dose of anti-VEGF until ME disappearance, then SDM within a month and, after that, anti-VEGF was delivered in PRN fashion.	BCVA: significant improvement from 0.52 $\pm$ 0.34 logMAR to 0.41 $\pm$ 0.34 logMAR at 12 months; stable reduction of CRT through 12 months from 491.1 $\pm$ 133.9 µm to 354.8 $\pm$ 120.4 µm; mean number of injections: 3.6 $\pm$ 2.1 during one year.

SDM, subthreshold diode micropulsation; IVR, intravitreal ranibizumab; IVA, intravitreal aflibercept; IVT, intravitreal triamcinolone; BCVA, best-corrected visual acuity; CRT, central retinal thickness; ME, macular edema; BRVO, branch retinal vein occlusion; DME, diabetic macular edema; CS, contrast sensitivity; ETDRS—Early Treatment Diabetic Retinopathy Study, RCT, randomized clinical trial; PRN, pro re nata. *, Manufactured by Allergan, Dublin, Ireland.

The triamcinolone study in ME secondary to BRVO clearly favored combined intravitreal triamcinolone (IVT) + SDM therapy over SDM alone [15]. Those patients who were subjected to combined treatment achieved better functional results than those who received SDM monotherapy. In the DME study of similar design, both the combined therapy and SDM-alone protocols proved equally effective in maintaining initial BCVA and improving retinal morphology; however, it should be remembered that baseline retinal thickness was significantly less in the SDM-alone group [16].

In the study by Elhamid et al., SDM was performed one month after intravitreal Ozurdex injection (Allergan, Dublin, Ireland) in patients with DME resistant to anti-VEGF therapy [17]. Although the results suggested the occurrence of significant morphological and functional improvements, the trial did not include a control group, so it was not possible to assess how the addition of SDM to intravitreal dexamethasone affected the final outcome. A study by Inagaki et al., which considered SDM and anti-VEGF therapy in DME is a case series, [18] observed a moderate BCVA improvement (by 0.11 logMAR), with a relatively low number of injections required to achieve this effect during one year of follow-up (mean: 3.6 ± 2.1 injections).

4. Discussion

Literature material for the analysis of the efficacy of the combination of SDM and intravitreal treatment in DME and RVO is scarce. Following a search of PubMed, only five eligible comparative studies were identified, including two randomized trials. Some collective findings from these studies can be reported and analyzed, although caution must be maintained. Generally, patients subjected to combined therapy required fewer injections, especially when this number was compared with the number of anti-VEGF treatments in the monotherapy population. If this outcome is confirmed in larger studies, SDM could be adopted in clinical practice to significantly reduce the burden of the treatment of retinal vascular diseases both financially and with respect to the patient's comfort.

From the available material, it was determined that combined treatment was not inferior to anti-VEGF therapy alone when considering improvements in BCVA and retinal morphology. However, SDM was usually performed in cases of minor and moderate retinal edema or following the resolution of edema after a loading dose of the intravitreal injection was delivered. This is consistent with the results of other research correlating SDM efficacy with the amount of baseline ME, often suggesting a central retinal thickness of 400 μm as the threshold [19–21]. This fact implicates a strict rationale is necessary during combined SDM and anti-VEGF treatment in that the adjunct of SDM is only sensible in cases with less severe retinal edema or following a reduction in edema prompted by initial anti-VEGF therapy.

Unfortunately, the analysis of the material does not offer us a precise answer regarding what should be the treatment schedule for the combined therapy. Both the number of loading-phase injections and the moment of SDM application varied among the studies. Further research needs to address the following questions that remain: what is the optimal number of injections required during the loading phase of intravitreal therapy, what is the best time point of SDM application (e.g., complete resolution of ME, reduction below 400 μm, or reference to BCVA), and what is the ideal the retreatment schedule for either anti-VEGF or SDM? Some form of an algorithm for combined treatment in DME has already been proposed, yet it is not backed by published research [22]. SDM or anti-VEGF was suggested as the first-line therapy for DME of less than 250 μm. For larger cases of edema, an initial loading phase of two to three anti-VEGF injections followed by three injections in the context of a good response is recommended. Thereafter, switching to SDM is suggested. However, if the response is poor after two or three initial injections, a switch to SDM earlier on is indicated. Luttrull et al. does not use retinal thickness as a signal for deciding how to treat DME; if the VA is 20/50 or worse, an initial anti-VEGF injection is given and injections are continued until the VA is 20/40 or better, at which time panmacular SDM is initiated (there is no loading dose custom), while, if the VA is 20/40 or better, SDM is performed alone [23].

This review also discusses a number of non-comparative studies that do not directly refer the combined treatment to intravitreal therapy alone (Table 2). As the literature on the subject was really limited, the author attempted to evaluate each study that reported effects of combination treatment that included SDM. Two studies presented in Table 2 provide some perspective on the position of combination therapy, including SDM versus SDM alone [15,16]. It seems that SDM works well alone in mild to moderate DME; however, there is a tendency for better morphological results to be obtained with the involvement of intravitreal medication [16]. In BRVO, an additive strong anti-inflammatory effect of intravitreal steroids provided significant improvements that were clearly superior to SDM only [15]. The remaining two studies reported an effect of SDM added to either intravitreal steroid or anti-VEGF therapy in the treatment of DME [17,18]. The lack of a control groups in these reports makes their interpretation rather risky and, despite favorable morphological and functional outcomes, the benefit of adding SDM to the treatment regimen is impossible to evaluate. Moreover, it must be emphasized that intravitreal steroid therapy in the treatment of DME and ME secondary to BRVO in most cases remains the second line of therapy, as does its combination with SDM.

The author realizes that the scarceness of literature on combined treatment including both SDM and intravitreal therapy for ME does not allow for a systematic review to be performed nor for the presentation of concrete conclusions. However, in the author's opinion, this limitation only means that this form of treatment should be looked at more carefully. The common use of intravitreal injections—anti-VEGF in particular—has pushed aside other forms of treatment, some of which are potentially effective. SDM is rarely given attention by members of industry, who support multicenter clinical trials. Thus, designing and carrying out a large SDM investigation including numerous cases is not easy and requires a lot of perseverance. Reviews such as this one will hopefully stimulate researchers to pursue the subject further.

5. Conclusions

An analysis of the available research on combined SDM and anti-VEGF/intravitreal treatment in ME does not provide an unequivocal answer at this time regarding the efficacy and benefits of this clinical approach. Existing published results suggest that combining SDM and anti-VEGF in the treatment of cases of limited retinal edema would reduce the number of intravitreal injections required, with functional and morphological outcomes that are non-inferior to those of anti-VEGF monotherapy. Larger, randomized clinical trials are needed to confirm this thesis and provide a rational treatment algorithm.

Funding: No funding was received for this research.

Institutional Review Board Statement: Not applicable (the study is a systemized review).

Informed Consent Statement: Not applicable (the study is a systemized review).

Data Availability Statement: No new data were created or analyzed in this study. Data sharing is not applicable to this article.

Conflicts of Interest: The author declares no conflict of interest.

Ethical Statement: This study was approved by the Dobry Wzrok Ophthalmological Clinic committee.

References

1. Gawęcki, M. Micropulse Laser Treatment of Retinal Diseases. *J. Clin. Med.* **2019**, *8*, 242. [CrossRef]
2. Brader, H.S.; Young, L.H.Y. Subthreshold Diode Micropulse Laser: A Review. *Semin. Ophthalmol.* **2016**, *31*, 30–39. [CrossRef] [PubMed]
3. Gawęcki, M.; Jaszczuk-Maciejewska, A.; Jurska-Jaśko, A.; Kneba, M.; Grzybowski, A. Transfoveal Micropulse Laser Treatment of Central Serous Chorioretinopathy within Six Months of Disease Onset. *J. Clin. Med.* **2019**, *8*, 1398. [CrossRef]
4. Luttrull, J.K. Low-intensity/high-density subthreshold diode micropulse laser for central serous chorioretinopathy. *Retin.* **2016**, *36*, 1658–1663. [CrossRef]
5. Scholz, P.; Ersoy, L.; Boon, C.J.; Fauser, S. Subthreshold Micropulse Laser (577 nm) Treatment in Chronic Central Serous Chorioretinopathy. *Ophthalmologica* **2015**, *234*, 189–194. [CrossRef]
6. Scholz, P.; Altay, L.; Fauser, S. A Review of Subthreshold Micropulse Laser for Treatment of Macular Disorders. *Adv. Ther.* **2017**, *34*, 1528–1555. [CrossRef]
7. Ciulla, T.A.; Bracha, P.; Pollack, J.; Williams, D.F. Real-world Outcomes of Anti–Vascular Endothelial Growth Factor Therapy in Diabetic Macular Edema in the United States. *Ophthalmol. Retin.* **2018**, *2*, 1179–1187. [CrossRef]
8. Korobelnik, J.-F.; Daien, V.; Faure, C.; Tadayoni, R.; Giocanti-Auregan, A.; Dot, C.; Kodjikian, L.; Massin, P. Real-world outcomes following 12 months of intravitreal aflibercept monotherapy in patients with diabetic macular edema in France: Results from the APOLLON study. *Graefe Arch. Clin. Exp. Ophthalmol.* **2020**, *258*, 521–528. [CrossRef]
9. Gross, J.G.; Glassman, A.R.; Liu, D.; Sun, J.K.; Antoszyk, A.N.; Baker, C.W.; Bressler, N.M.; Elman, M.J.; Ferris, F.L.; Gardner, T.W.; et al. Five-year outcomes of panretinal photocoagulation vs. intravitreous ranibizumab for proliferative diabetic retinopathy: A randomized clinical trial. *JAMA Ophthalmol.* **2018**, *136*, 1138–1148. [PubMed]

10. Thinda, S.; Patel, A.; Hunter, A.A.; Moshiri, A.; Morse, L.S. Combination therapy with subthreshold diode laser micropulse photocoagulation and intravitreal anti-vascular endothelial growth factor injections for diabetic macular edema. *Invest. Ophthalmol. Vis. Sci.* **2014**, *55*, 6363.
11. Moisseiev, E.; Abbassi, S.; Thinda, S.; Yoon, J.; Yiu, G.; Morse, L.S. Subthreshold micropulse laser reduces anti-VEGF injection burden in patients with diabetic macular edema. *Eur. J. Ophthalmol.* **2018**, *28*, 68–73. [CrossRef]
12. Khattab, A.M.; Hagras, S.M.; Abdelhamid, A.; Torky, M.A.; Awad, E.A.; Abdelhameed, A.G. Aflibercept with adjuvant micropulsed yellow laser versus aflibercept monotherapy in diabetic macular edema. *Graefe Arch. Clin. Exp. Ophthalmol.* **2019**, *257*, 1373–1380. [CrossRef]
13. Kanar, H.S.; Arsan, A.; Altun, A.; Akı, S.F.; Hacısalihoglu, A. Can subthreshold micropulse yellow laser treatment change the antivascular endothelial growth factor algorithm in diabetic macular edema? A randomized clinical trial. *Indian J. Ophthalmol.* **2020**, *68*, 145–151. [PubMed]
14. Terashima, H.; Hasebe, H.; Okamoto, F.; Matsuoka, N.; Sato, Y.; Fukuchi, T. Combination therapy of intravitreal ranibizumab and subthreshold micropulse photocoagulation for macular edema secondary to branch retinal vein occlusion: 6-month result. *Retina* **2019**, *39*, 1377–1384. [CrossRef]
15. Parodi, M.B.; Iacono, P.; Ravalico, G. Intravitreal triamcinolone acetonide combined with subthreshold grid laser treatment for macular oedema in branch retinal vein occlusion: A pilot study. *Br. J. Ophthalmol.* **2008**, *92*, 1046–1050. [CrossRef] [PubMed]
16. Luttrull, J.K.; Sramek, C.; Palanker, D.; Spink, C.J.; Musch, D.C. Long-term safety, high-resolution imaging, and tissue temperature modeling of subvisible diode micropulse photocoagulation for retinovascular macular edema. *Retina* **2012**, *32*, 375–386. [CrossRef]
17. Elhamid, A.H.A. Combined intravitreal dexamethasone implant and micropulse yellow laser for treatment of anti-VEGF re-sistant diabetic macular edema. *Open Ophthalmol. J.* **2017**, *11*, 164–172. [CrossRef]
18. Inagaki, K.; Hamada, M.; Ohkoshi, K. Minimally invasive laser treatment combined with intravitreal injection of anti-vascular endothelial growth factor for diabetic macular oedema. *Sci. Rep.* **2019**, *9*, 1–8. [CrossRef]
19. Midena, E.; Bini, S.; Martini, F.; Enrica, C.; Pilotto, E.; Micera, A.; Esposito, G.; Vujosevic, S. Changes of aqueous humor müller cells' biomarkers in human patients affected by diabetic macular edema after subthreshold micropulse laser treatment. *Retina* **2020**, *40*, 126–134. [CrossRef]
20. Mansouri, A.; Sampat, K.M.; Malik, K.J.; Steiner, J.N.; Glaser, B.M. Efficacy of subthreshold micropulse laser in the treatment of diabetic macular edema is influenced by pre-treatment central foveal thickness. *Eye* **2014**, *28*, 1418–1424. [CrossRef] [PubMed]
21. Vujosevic, S.; Martini, F.; Longhin, E.; Convento, E.; Cavarzeran, F.; Midena, E. Subthreshold micropulse yellow laser versus subthreshold micropulse infrared laser in center-involving diabetic macular edema: Morphologic and functional safety. *Retina* **2015**, *35*, 1594–1603. [CrossRef] [PubMed]
22. Mansour, S.; Luttrull, J. Integration of Micro Pulse Laser Therapy (MPLT) in the Management of Diabetic Retinopathy; IRIDEX Educational Webinar. 2012. Available online: http://www.iridex.com.
23. Luttrull, J.K. SDM as Modern Retinal Laser Therapy. Principles, Practice and RWD. Available online: https://www.researchgate.net/project/SDM-as-Modern-Retinal-Laser-Therapy-Principles-Practice-and-RWD (accessed on 20 January 2021).

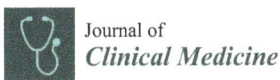

Review

Treatment of Macular Edema in Vascular Retinal Diseases: A 2021 Update

Andrzej Grzybowski [1,2], Agne Markeviciute [3] and Reda Zemaitiene [3,*]

1. Department of Ophthalmology, University of Warmia and Mazury, 10-561 Olsztyn, Poland; ae.grzybowski@gmail.com
2. Institute for Research in Ophthalmology, 60-836 Poznan, Poland
3. Department of Ophthalmology, Medical Academy, Lithuanian University of Health Sciences, 50161 Kaunas, Lithuania; markeviciutee.agne@gmail.com
* Correspondence: reda.zemaitiene@lsmuni.lt

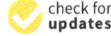

Citation: Grzybowski, A.; Markeviciute, A.; Zemaitiene, R. Treatment of Macular Edema in Vascular Retinal Diseases: A 2021 Update. *J. Clin. Med.* **2021**, *10*, 5300. https://doi.org/10.3390/jcm10225300

Academic Editors: Gawęcki Maciej and Stephen Andrew Vernon

Received: 11 August 2021
Accepted: 11 November 2021
Published: 15 November 2021

Publisher's Note: MDPI stays neutral with regard to jurisdictional claims in published maps and institutional affiliations.

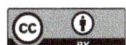

Copyright: © 2021 by the authors. Licensee MDPI, Basel, Switzerland. This article is an open access article distributed under the terms and conditions of the Creative Commons Attribution (CC BY) license (https://creativecommons.org/licenses/by/4.0/).

Abstract: Macular edema (ME) is associated with various conditions; however, the main causes of ME are retinal vein occlusion (RVO) and diabetes. Laser photocoagulation, formerly the gold standard for the treatment of ME, has been replaced by anti-vascular endothelial growth factor (anti-VEGF) intravitreal injections. Despite its efficiency, this treatment requires frequent injections to preserve the outcomes of anti-VEGF therapy, and as many patients do not sufficiently respond to the treatment, ME is typically a chronic condition that can lead to permanent visual impairment. Generalized recommendations for the treatment of ME are lacking, which highlights the importance of reviewing treatment approaches, including recent anti-VEGFs, intravitreal steroid implants, and subthreshold micropulse lasers. We reviewed relevant studies, emphasizing the articles published between 2019 and 2021 and using the following keywords: macular edema, diabetic macular edema, retinal vein occlusion, laser photocoagulation, anti-VEGF, and intravitreal injections. Our results revealed that a combination of different treatment methods may be beneficial in resistant cases. Additionally, artificial intelligence (AI) is likely to help select the best treatment option for patients in the near future.

Keywords: macular edema; diabetic macular edema; retinal vein occlusion; laser photocoagulation; anti-VEGF; intravitreal injections

1. Introduction

Macular edema (ME) is a disease characterized by the swelling of the macula due to the abnormal accumulation of fluid [1]. It is associated with increased macular thickness and significantly reduced visual acuity, and it may develop in various ocular conditions.

Postoperative cystoid macular edema (PCME) typically occurs after cataract surgery; however, it can occur after any ocular surgery [2]. The increased phacoemulsification energy and phacoemulsification time or postoperative pseudophakodonesis can significantly contribute to PCME development [3]. It is thought that topical prostaglandin analogs used for glaucoma treatment may also promote PCME [3,4].

Corticosteroid eyedrops are prescribed postoperatively by most cataract surgeons to prevent the formation of PCME [5]. Topical steroids, non-steroidal anti-inflammatory eye drops, and ocular steroid injections (sub-tenon or intravitreal) are the main treatment options for PCME [2].

ME is the most common cause of vision loss in patients with uveitis [6,7]. Although both regional and systemic steroids are considered effective treatments, other treatment options are available, including immunomodulatory agents and anti-vascular endothelial growth factor (VEGF) intravitreal injections [7,8].

Cystoid macular edema (CME) is observed in patients with various retinal pathologies. It is considered a complication in patients with retinitis pigmentosa (RP), whereas tractional CME is associated with the persistent attachment of the vitreous at the macular region [9,10].

However, in most eyes undergoing treatment of ME related to retinal vascular disease, it is diabetic macular edema (DME) and retinal vein occlusion (RVO) that are the driving forces.

ME affects approximately 7 million patients with diabetic retinopathy (DR) and 3 million patients with retinal vein occlusion (RVO) [11].

The role of inherited genetic polymorphisms in DME development and treatment response is still poorly understood; nevertheless, possible DME risk genes have been identified. Graham and colleagues did not find any significant genome-wide associations with DME risk; however, they identified the top-ranked single nucleotide polymorphism (SNP) for DME in rs1990145 on chromosome 2 [12]. A trend toward an association between DME and DR was detected in two SNPs: rs12267418, near *MALRD1* ($p = 0.008$), and rs16999051 in the diabetes gene *PCSK2* ($p = 0.007$) [12,13]. It is clear that there is a need for larger studies.

CME involves fluid accumulation in the outer plexiform layer of the retina due to abnormal perifoveal retinal capillary permeability, whereas DME is associated with the leakage of macular capillaries and is observed in patients suffering from diabetes [14]. ME is also associated with an increase in VEGF and interleukin 6, which induce vascular permeability and vasodilation [15].

Chronic ME leads to permanent visual impairment by altering the outer limiting membrane, affecting photoreceptor segments (outer nuclear layer thinning and outer segment atrophy), and disorganization of inner retinal layers [11].

ME treatment approaches have changed substantially in recent years. Although laser photocoagulation (LP) has long been the gold standard for the treatment of ME, it is being replaced by anti-VEGF intravitreal injections, which have been reported as a first-line treatment for both DME and ME due to RVO.

This paper reviews and analyzes recent approaches to ME treatment and discusses future directions and perspectives in this field.

2. Methodology

A search of the medical literature was performed in PubMed and Google Scholar up to April 2021. The following keywords were used in various combinations: macular edema, diabetic macular edema, retinal vein occlusion, Laser Photocoagulation, anti-VEGF, intravitreal injections, and uveitis. Only articles with English abstracts focusing on ME caused by retinal vascular diseases, including DME and ME due to RVO, were reviewed. Studies were critically reviewed to construct an overview and guidance for further searches and highlight the lack of generalized recommendations. Emphasis was placed on articles published between 2019 and 2021.

3. Results

Intravitreal ranibizumab and aflibercept are currently approved for ME treatment, whereas bevacizumab is used off-label, and conbercept is approved and used for DME treatment only in China [16]. Frequent injections are required to preserve the effects of anti-VEGF therapy, and this treatment is therefore associated with repeated risk, high costs and an increasing burden on ophthalmologists and their patients. Despite the reported efficacy of anti-VEGFs, many patients do not respond well to treatment. In addition, identifying which treatment regimen is optimal is a constant dilemma. The main advantage of treat-and-extend (T and E) over pro re nata (PRN) regimens is a reduction in the number of hospital visits and recurrences [17]. Elsebaey and colleagues compared T and E treatment regimen with the PRN regimen in patients with DME [18]. They concluded that an individualized T and E regimen has the potential to reduce the clinic burden and improve patient compliance while maintaining effectiveness and providing well-tolerated treatment for DME [18]. Similar results were reported by Kim et al.: the T and E regimen of aflibercept in DME maintained effectiveness in a 2-year follow-up and reduced the number of injections compared with fixed dosing regimens [17].

Intravitreal corticosteroid implants ensure sustained drug release for a specific period and reduce the number of injections needed compared with anti-VEGF treatment. Steroid implants were reported to be effective and safe both in DME and ME due to RVO; however, they are typically used as a second choice in cases resistant to anti-VEGF treatment. The intravitreal dexamethasone (DEX) implant is approved for the treatment of DME and ME due to RVO; in the EU, it is approved for use in patients with DME that responds poorly to other treatments and for those who are pseudophakic or ineligible for other therapies [19]. The fluocinolone acetonide (FA) implant is approved for the treatment of DME and is typically used in patients who previously received a course of corticosteroids and did not experience a significant increase in eye pressure [20]. Despite the efficacy of steroids, they may be associated with increased intraocular pressure (IOP) and cataract formation.

Resistance to anti-VEGFs and intravitreal steroids treatment methods highlights the need for alternative treatment options.

3.1. Diabetic Macular Edema

The main DME treatment options are intravitreal injections of anti-VEGF agents and intravitreal corticosteroid injections. Formerly, macular LP was the gold standard for DME treatment; however, it is now utilized as an additional treatment. The two most common techniques of LP in patients with DME are focal photocoagulation targeting focal lesions (e.g., leaking microaneurysms or ischemic areas on fluorescein angiography (FA) for focal DME cases) and the grid laser technique, in which the laser is applied to diffuse leakages or nonperfusion areas; the latter is recommended for diffuse or more severe forms of DME [21,22]. According to the European Society of Retina Specialists (EURETINA) guidelines published in 2017, the focal and grid laser techniques should be utilized for non-center involving DME [23]. The laser can reportedly be applied in the vasogenic subform of DME, which is clinically characterized by the presence of focally grouped microaneurysms (MA) and leaking capillaries [24]. The primary reason grid laser is not recommended further is because of retinal scarring; however, when targeting capillary microaneurysms, a focal laser is beneficial as a second-line treatment [24,25]. In addition, it can be considered as a combined treatment option to reduce the number of anti-VEGF injections. Paques and colleagues performed a pilot study and reported significantly reduced macular thickness and improved visual acuity after elective photocoagulation of capillary microaneurysms in patients with chronic macular edema and severe hard exudates due to diabetic retinopathy or RVO [26].

Most studies found anti-VEGFs to be superior to laser treatment in DME patients. The REFINE study was conducted in Chinese patients with DME who received intravitreal ranibizumab injections or LP [27]. The results revealed a significantly greater improvement in mean best-corrected visual acuity (BCVA) at month 12 with ranibizumab than with LP [27]. Singh and colleagues reported that BCVA improvement was significantly greater with aflibercept than with laser techniques and was not influenced by any baseline factors [28,29]. A subthreshold micropulse laser (SML) is a relatively new tissue-sparing laser technique; it avoids protein coagulation and prevents retinal scars, allowing the preservation of retinal anatomy and function [30].

SML helps improve or stabilize visual function and decrease macular thickness in DME [31]. Vujosevic and colleagues performed a study that evaluated the effectiveness of SML treatment in patients with DME [31]. They reported that 31 patients (83.8%) required retreatment (mean number of SML treatments over 12 months: 2.19 ± 0.7); however, no eyes needed any additional treatments (anti-VEGF, steroids, and/or conventional laser) [31]. Al-Barki et al. compared the outcomes between short-pulse continuous wavelength and infrared micropulse lasers in DME treatment [32]. The authors concluded that the infrared micropulse system improved functional outcomes in patients with DME, whereas the short-pulse system resulted in a greater temporary reduction in edema [32].

Gawęcki and colleagues performed a systematized review and proposed that combining the SML treatment with anti-VEGFs may require fewer intravitreal injections than anti-VEGF monotherapy with equally favorable functional and morphological results in the ME treatment. However, SML alone was not superior to intravitreal treatment alone or combined treatment [33]. The authors noted that the studies under review varied in treatment protocols and inclusion criteria [33]. Altinel and colleagues compared the efficacy and safety of SML and intravitreal bevacizumab (IVB) injection combined therapy with IVB monotherapy in DME treatment [34]. They concluded that fewer IVB injections were needed when laser treatment was added; however, a significant increase in BCVA was not achieved [34]. Similarly, Furashova et al. reported that patients treated with ranibizumab combined with additional laser treatment experienced greater visual improvement and required fewer ranibizumab injections compared with patients treated only with ranibizumab [35].

Valera-Cornejo et al. evaluated the effect of SML treatment in center-involved DME in previously untreated (naïve) patients and patients who did not respond to prior treatment [36]. No significant changes in BCVA were observed between the groups after 3 months [36]. The change in central macular thickness (CMT) at 3 months was statistically but not clinically significant in the treatment-naïve group only, and no adverse events were reported [36]. Passos et al. reported that SML treatment used alone was not as effective as it could be when combined with other treatments [37]. DME cases associated with subretinal fluid had the best anatomical response, whereas intraretinal edema responded poorly to laser monotherapy [37]. The authors concluded that SML might be used in a combination treatment for ME [37]. Other authors also suggest considering laser therapy as an additional treatment in combination with intravitreal injections [21].

Anti-VEGFs utilize different molecules to achieve their effect: aptamers (pegaptanib); antibodies to VEGF (bevacizumab); antibody fragments to VEGF (ranibizumab); and fusion proteins, which combine a receptor for VEGF with the constant region of a human immunoglobulin (aflibercept and conbercept) [28]. Bevacizumab, ranibizumab, and aflibercept are the most common anti-VEGFs, and many studies have not observed significant differences in outcomes between them [28,38]. However, it has been suggested that the choice of anti-VEGF can be guided by the untreated BCVA. When it is lower, aflibercept has been suggested as the drug of choice [28,29]. The remaining anti-VEGFs, including bevacizumab, ranibizumab, and aflibercept, provide similar functional outcomes when the baseline BCVA is higher [28]. Bressler and colleagues, however, reported that after six consecutive injections, more patients presented with persistent ME following bevacizumab treatment compared with ranibizumab and aflibercept [39]. On this basis, Haritoglou et al. suggested switching from bevacizumab to either aflibercept or ranibizumab if DME persists while using bevacizumab [40].

Zhou et al. evaluated the efficacy and safety of intravitreal conbercept for DME treatment [41]. Patients were treated with one to three consecutive monthly intravitreal conbercept (IVC) injections, followed by retreatment with conbercept or switch therapy with triamcinolone acetonide (TA) based on a 6-month observation of the effect of treatment [29]. Approximately one-third of the eyes (29 of 89 eyes involved in the study) received intravitreal triamcinolone acetonide (IVTA) injections at month 6 [41]. The results revealed that the mean BCVA and CMT were significantly improved at 1 and 3 months after IVC treatment in the IVC group, and they gradually improved at 9 months after IVTA treatments in the IVC plus IVTA group [41]. Five eyes exhibited aggravated cataracts at the last follow-up visit after IVTA injection, and this was associated with the final decline in BCVA [41]. Nonetheless, the authors concluded that conbercept is safe and efficient, and TA may be beneficial in cases that are refractory to anti-VEGF treatment [41]. A meta-analysis comparing the efficacies of conbercept and ranibizumab for DME treatment demonstrated that intravitreal conbercept was significantly superior to ranibizumab in reducing CMT; however, no significant difference in visual improvement was observed [42]. The effects and safety of conbercept and ranibizumab in DME treatment were also compared in a recent meta-analysis by Sun et al., and the results demonstrated that intravitreal injections of conbercept were superior to ranibizumab in both reducing central retinal thickness and improving BCVA [43].

Corticosteroids are typically used as an alternative therapy for eyes with an insufficient response to anti-VEGF treatment reducing inflammation, decreasing the disruption of the blood–retinal barrier, and interfering with retinal angiogenesis [44]. Although intravitreal steroids are not used as often as anti-VEGFs, they can significantly reduce DME, and some authors suggest them as an option for first-line treatment. The main steroids used for the treatment of DME are TA, dexamethasone (DEX), and FA, which differ in their duration of action [40]. Because of the short vitreous elimination half-life of the solubilized fraction of these steroids, an extended duration of action can be achieved by applying sustained release systems (implants) into the vitreous cavity [40]. After one intravitreal injection of TA, the treatment effect was maintained for up to 6 months [40]. However, TA elevates the risk of increased IOP, and it may be associated with the risk of pseudoendophthalmitis [45,46] and retinal toxicity [47–49]; thus, it is used less frequently than its alternatives [40]. Additionally, TA has not been approved for DME treatment [28]. Conversely, the DEX drug release injectable implant has higher recognition, with a pharmacological effect ranging between 4 and 6 months [40].

A first-line treatment algorithm and guidelines in center-involving DME have been suggested by Kodjikian et al. [50]. The authors included a slow-release 700 µg dexamethasone intravitreal implant as an option for first-line treatment in center-involving DME, together with three anti-VEGFs (bevacizumab, ranibizumab, and aflibercept). Augustin and colleagues reported a consensus by a group of retina experts indicating that if a patient does not exhibit a sufficient response after 3–6 months of anti-VEGF treatment (a visual acuity gain of <5 ETDRS letters or a reduction in the central retinal thickness of ≤20%), switching to the dexamethasone implant should be considered [51]. An implant may also be suitable in eyes with massive lipid exudates or as a first-line treatment in pseudophakic patients, patients unwilling or unable to comply with tight anti-VEGF injection intervals, or patients with known vascular diseases [51].

Intravitreal DEX implants were reported to be effective in cases that were refractory to anti-VEGF treatment. Castro-Navarro and colleagues reported that the intravitreal DEX implant was effective and safe in both previously treated and untreated patients with DME [52]. Additionally, the authors observed that 6 months after the injection of the DEX implant, patients without prior DME treatment gained significantly more letters than patients who were previously treated [52]. These results suggest the possibility of achieving better results with earlier DEX implantation. This agrees with the results of a study by Medina-Baena, which demonstrated that at month 12, naïve patients exhibited a greater improvement in BCVA from baseline and achieved this BCVA improvement significantly faster than previously treated patients [53]. Similar results were observed in a study by Iglicki et al. [54]. They found that over a follow-up of 24 months, the vision in DME eyes improved after treatment with DEX implants in eyes that were treatment-naïve and in eyes that were refractory to anti-VEGF treatment; however, a greater improvement was observed in naïve eyes [54].

Although most studies evaluate CMT as the target of anatomical outcomes, Altun and colleagues evaluated the subfoveal choroidal thickness (SFCT) in vitrectomized eyes of patients with DME after intravitreal DEX implants [55]. The authors reported a statistically significant thinning of the mean SFCT during the follow-up period after DEX implant injection in vitrectomized eyes with DME [55].

Hong et al. performed a retrospective study to evaluate the effect of intravitreal TA injections in patients who were refractory to anti-VEGF treatment [44]. The authors reported that the BCVA improved significantly, and CMT was significantly reduced after a single TA intravitreal injection [44]. In addition, poorer visual acuity (VA) before the injection was associated with visual gain 1 month after the treatment [44]. Elevated IOP was observed in 17.1% of eyes, and this was observed significantly more often after IVTA injections containing a preservative than after preservative-free injections [39].

A longer pharmacological effect lasting up to 3 years can be achieved with an intravitreal FA sustained-release non-biodegradable device, which is inserted into the vitreous cavity via a 25-gauge needle; it contains 0.19 mg of FA and has a release rate of 0.2 µg/day [11]. Augustin and colleagues performed a retrospective study to evaluate the results of DME treatment with FA implants [56]. They concluded that a single FA implant could maintain reduced CMT for up to 3 years [56]. Several more studies reported similar results, highlighting that FA has a favorable safety and effectiveness profile while reducing CMT and improving BCVA [57–59]. Notably, Coelho and colleagues reported that FA exhibited long-term effectiveness in vitrectomized DME eyes and sustained the effectiveness in DME eyes that did not respond to DEX therapy [60].

The correct time to switch therapy if patients do not respond to anti-VEGF treatment remains unclear. Gonzalez et al. performed a study and reported that in eyes with poor responses after three anti-VEGF injections, it may be beneficial to switch to other modes of therapy [61]. Baker and colleagues found that for patients with DME and excellent visual acuity (defined as 20/25 or better), observation appeared to be a non-inferior initial management strategy compared with intravitreal aflibercept or LP in terms of visual acuity outcomes after 2 years [62]. Likewise, it was reported that initial focal or grid laser significantly reduced the risk of requiring aflibercept injection during follow-up [62].

Martínez and colleagues evaluated the effect of early DEX implantation in eyes with DME that received three or fewer anti-VEGF injections before the switch as well as the effect of later implantation in patients who received six or more anti-VEGF injections before the switch [63]. They reported that an early switch to DEX in patients who did not adequately respond to anti-VEGF therapy provided better results: BCVA improved significantly more (compared with baseline), and CMT decreased more in the early switch group compared with the late switch group [63]. In addition, no difference in the incidence of increased IOP was observed between the groups [63]. Comparable results were reported in Demir and colleagues' study; the authors concluded that the central retinal thickness (CRT) decreased significantly more in the early switch group compared with the later switch group [64]. These results agree with those of a study by Ruiz-Medrano et al. [45]. Superior functional outcomes were observed in eyes with insufficient responses to anti-VEGFs in patients switched to DEX who had been receiving three monthly anti-VEGF injections compared with those who had been receiving more than three monthly anti-VEGF injections [65].

Cataract surgery can induce DME progression as well as the development of DME in patients with diabetes [28]. Several studies have reported improved functional and anatomic clinical outcomes in patients with DEX implants during cataract surgery [66–68]. Furino and colleagues conducted a study to evaluate functional and anatomical outcomes after combined phacoemulsification and intravitreal DEX implantation with standard phacoemulsification in diabetic patients with cataracts [69]. In the group with combined phacoemulsification and intravitreal DEX implantation, BCVA improved significantly more, and central subfoveal thickness decreased more [69]. Although this group had significantly higher IOP during follow-up at month 3 compared with baseline, IOP remained within the normal range [69].

Possibilities for future treatment include ziv-aflibercept, which was proposed as a new recombinant fusion protein and which has a mechanism of action similar to that of aflibercept; however, it is available at a lower cost than the proprietary anti-VEGF drug [70]. It was reported to be effective and safe in DME treatment and other retinal diseases; however, further studies are needed [70,71]. Because of the longer intravitreal half-life of the new generation anti-VEGF-A inhibitors, including brolucizumab, abicipar pegol, and angiopoietin combination drugs, improved prolonged edema reduction and less frequent injections appear to be required [11,28]. The preliminary results of studies currently in progress have suggested that anti-VEGF-A may have superior effectiveness compared with approved anti-VEGFs [11,28,72].

Rivera et al. reported evidence of reduction of DME through the consumption of lutein. In patients with ME who have lower levels of lutein, lutein consumption prevented and reduced possible complications [73].

A summary of the treatment options for DME is presented in Table 1.

Table 1. Summary of treatment of diabetic macular edema.

	Considered First-Line Treatment	Insufficient Response to Anti-VEGF	
DME	Intravitreal anti-VEGF injections ○ Bevacizumab, ranibizumab, and aflibercept are the most used anti-VEGFs, and many studies have not identified significant differences in outcomes between them ○ The choice of one anti-VEGF over another depends on baseline BCVA	Intravitreal steroid (DEX/FA) implants ○ Sustained drug release for a specific period ○ Acts on different targets than anti-VEGF agents by reducing inflammation, decreasing the disruption of the blood–retinal barrier, and interfering with retinal angiogenesis ○ A slow-release 700 µg dexamethasone intravitreal implant can be considered as an option for first-line treatment in center-involving DME ○ DEX can be considered as first-line therapy in pseudophakic patients without advanced or uncontrolled glaucoma ○ FA can be considered in pseudophakic patients in whom DEX has been well-tolerated ○ * TA—has not been approved for DME	Micropulse laser therapy/ conventional focal laser therapy ○ Helps improve or stabilize visual function and decrease the macular thickness ○ Can reduce the number of intravitreal injections when used as a combined treatment

DEX—dexamethasone, DME—diabetic macular edema, BCVA—best corrected visual acuity, FA—fluocinolone acetonide, VEGF—vascular endothelial growth factor, TA—triamcinolone acetonide, * not an approved treatment.

3.2. Macular Edema Secondary to Retinal Vein Occlusion

Retinal vein occlusion (RVO) includes branch RVO (BRVO), central RVO (CRVO), and hemi-RVO, which are categorized according to the anatomic location of the occlusion [74]. In all hemorrhages and ME occur, leading to significant visual impairment [75].

Although LP has long been considered a primary treatment option, similar to DME, it has been replaced by other treatment methods. It was reported that although macular grid laser treatment reduced vision loss and the risk of vitreous hemorrhage in eyes with ME due to BRVO, it was ineffective against ME due to CRVO [15,74]. Zhang and colleagues additionally reported that LP cannot be performed in cases of retinal swelling with hemorrhage because the laser energy is absorbed and reduced; however, laser therapy may be used as rescue therapy for ME secondary to RVO [74].

Hayreh et al. has reported that in patients with ME due to RVO who respond poorly to anti-VEGF therapy or are incapable or reluctant to attend clinics for frequent anti-VEGF injections, grid laser treatment can be used combined with anti-VEGF therapy [76].

Intravitreal anti-VEGF injections are now considered the first-line treatment for ME associated with RVO, and their efficacy and superiority over other treatment methods have been demonstrated in many studies. Qian et al.'s meta-analysis reported that anti-VEGFs were the most effective therapy for ME secondary to both CRVO and BRVO [77]. The survey study, which was performed among retina specialists in Japan, revealed that anti-VEGF therapy was chosen as the first-line treatment for ME secondary to BRVO, and most specialists (82.4%) selected initial injection followed by a pro re nata (PRN) regimen; however, the opinions about the initiation and switching therapy varied between specialists [78]. As additional treatment in refractory cases, laser therapy was reported as the most common choice (35.9%), with 25.6% selecting vitrectomy, and 15.4% chosing to add steroid injections [78].

Anti-VEGFs used to treat ME due to RVO are similar to those used to treat DME; ranibizumab and aflibercept are used on label, whereas bevacizumab and conbercept have been used off label. Hykin and colleagues performed a prospective study to evaluate the effectiveness of ranibizumab, aflibercept, and bevacizumab for the management of ME due to CRVO [16]. They reported that mean changes in vision after 100 weeks of follow-up and treatment were not inferior with aflibercept than with ranibizumab; however, the mean number of injections given in the aflibercept group was lower than that in the ranibizumab group [16]. The mean changes in vision using bevacizumab compared with those using ranibizumab were similar, suggesting that the effectiveness of bevacizumab was neither equal nor superior to ranibizumab [16]. Conbercept is one of the newest anti-VEGFs and provided good treatment results in Chinese patients with RVO in a randomized clinical trial [79]. Xia and colleagues reported that conbercept significantly reduced retinal structural remodeling, inflammation, and oxidative stress in mice as well as in patients with ME due to RVO [75]. However, some patients with severe ME due to RVO did not experience significant benefit from conbercept [75]. The authors hypothesized that this may have been because conbercept only inhibits downstream VEGF inflammatory mediators and does not affect the upstream inflammatory mediators of VEGFs, such as PGE1, PGE2, and PGF2a [75]. Costa et al. reported that intravitreal anti-VEGF injections are prioritized over other treatment methods, including macular grid photocoagulation [80]. Compared with steroid injections, anti-VEGFs are superior because they have fewer side effects; as with their use in DME, steroids are associated with a higher incidence of increased IOP and cataract formation [80]. A systematic review and meta-analysis were performed by Liu and colleagues to evaluate the efficacy of conbercept and ranibizumab with or without LP in patients with ME secondary to RVO [81]. Both intravitreal conbercept and ranibizumab therapy with or without LP were effective in improving vision function in patients with ME secondary to RVO. The two anti-VEGFs did not differ significantly in BCVA improvement or adverse effects, and they resulted in similar visual gains [81]. However, conbercept reduced CMT more than ranibizumab with fewer injections [81]. Another systematic review performed by Spooner and colleagues evaluated 17 studies involving 1070 eyes [15]. It demonstrated that the management and outcomes of patients with CRVO varied greatly; however, anti-VEGF therapy significantly improved the anatomical and functional outcomes [15]. Although most eyes obtained a significant visual acuity gain, those treated with aflibercept and bevacizumab had significantly better outcomes than ranibizumab-treated eyes [15]. The incidence rates of ocular complications were low, including neovascular glaucoma (3.6%), vitreous hemorrhage (<1%), glaucoma (1.2%), and neovascular glaucoma (<1%) [15].

The management of cases refractory to anti-VEGF treatment is an ongoing dilemma, and therefore, the efficacy of steroids in patients with ME due to RVO has been explored in several studies. One study hypothesized that inflammation could be the first key mechanism to mechanical injury in RVO, and VEGF up-regulation may occur as a secondary effect of this inflammatory response [75]. Corticosteroids can significantly reduce inflammation, retinal vascular permeability, and the regulation of VEGF-A expression, and thus they have been used for the treatment of ME due to RVO [74]. The intravitreal dexamethasone implant is approved for the treatment of ME due to RVO [74]. Ming and colleagues performed a meta-analysis on the efficacy and safety of intravitreal DEX implants and anti-VEGFs for the treatment of ME due to RVO; the review included 4 randomized controlled trials and 12 real-world studies [19]. The authors reported that DEX implantation resulted in a comparable or smaller reduction in central subfield thickness (CST) at months 6 and 12 but introduced higher risks of elevated IOP and cataract induction [19]. It was concluded that compared with anti-VEGF agents, DEX implants required fewer injections but had inferior functional efficacy and safety [19].

The management of central and branch RVO and its long-term effects were evaluated in a 7-year follow-up study by Arrigo et al. performed in an Italian referral center [82]. Contrary to the previously discussed study, the authors reported that both CRVO and BRVO eyes exhibited significant visual acuity improvements secondary to intravitreal anti-VEGF or dexamethasone treatments and a significant reduction in CMT at the end of the follow-up. Furthermore, the authors highlighted a result that showed that the time at which the greatest improvement was observed differed between CRVO and BRVO; an earlier improvement was observed for CRVO (after 12 months of follow-up), and a later improvement was observed for BRVO (after 24 months of follow-up). However, after 2 years, both visual acuity and CMT remained stable until the end of follow-up.

Evidence of the value and importance of SML therapy in ME treatment is increasing. Buyru et al. compared the effects of intravitreal ranibizumab and SML treatment in two groups of patients with ME due to BRVO [83]. They concluded that the reduction in macular thickness and the increase in visual acuity were comparable for intravitreal ranibizumab and yellow SML treatment over 1 year. It was suggested that SML treatment may be useful in the treatment of ME due to BRVO. Eng and colleagues conducted a literature review on the efficacy of SML treatment for ME due to BRVO and reported that SML therapy resulted in a smaller reduction in ME compared with intravitreal anti-VEGF agents [84]. However, the authors concluded that SML treatment could be useful as adjuvant therapy with intravitreal anti-VEGF agents or steroids. Terashima et al. evaluated the efficacy of the combined therapy of intravitreal ranibizumab and 577 nm yellow laser SML photocoagulation for ME secondary to BRVO [85]. They concluded that combination therapy with intravitreal injections and SML was effective and decreased the frequency of intravitreal injections while maintaining good visual acuity. Similarly, a meta-analysis conducted by Chen et al. concluded that laser therapy combined with intravitreal ranibizumab injections had a strong effect, promoting its use for the treatment of ME secondary to BRVO in clinical practice [86].

Nanotechnology (nanocarriers) offers multiple benefits by promoting drug delivery across tissue barriers, controlling the release of a topically administered drug, improving bioavailability, and directing drugs to the target tissue [87]. An example of a nanosystem is the topical ophthalmic TA-loaded liposome formulation (TA-LF), which releases TA into the vitreous and retina [87]. It was reported to be safe and effective in rabbits as well as in patients with refractory pseudophakic cystoid ME. Navarro-Partida and colleagues evaluated its safety and efficacy in patients with ME secondary to BRVO who were given a topical instillation of one drop of TA-LF (TA 0.2%) six times a day for 12 weeks [87]. The results confirmed its effectiveness; a significant reduction in central foveal thickness and a significant improvement in BCVA were observed. No adverse events, including increased IOP, were reported. The authors suggested that as liposomes can function as nanocarriers of TA, they could allow topical ophthalmic therapy to become the primary treatment option instead of intravitreal drugs in patients with ME secondary to BRVO. Cheng et al.'s also showed that liposomes with TA in eye drops could be a new therapeutic approach for the effective treatment of retinal diseases [88].

Authors have investigated factors associated with the course of the disease and the response to the treatment. Kida and colleagues hypothesized that increased retinal venous pressure (RVP) plays an important role in the formation of macula edema; thus, they recently evaluated RVP before and 1 month after intravitreal ranibizumab injection to determine its effect on RVO-related ME [89]. They concluded that RVP decreased significantly after treatment; however, it remained significantly higher than the IOP. Rothman and colleagues assessed the impact of age on ME due to RVO and concluded that patients younger than 50 years old had higher baseline and final visual acuity, a lower incidence of cystoid macular edema at presentation, and received fewer intravitreal injections than older patients [90].

A summary of treatments for ME due to RVO is presented in Table 2.

Table 2. Summary of treatments for ME associated with RVO.

	First-line treatment	Cases resistant to anti-VEGF
ME associated with RVO	○ Intravitreal anti-VEGF injections ○ The superiority of agents in studies varies ○ Anti-VEGFs are chosen on the basis of baseline VA, drug price, and availability	○ Intravitreal steroid (DEX) implant ○ SML/conventional focal laser therapy as combined therapy

DEX—dexamethasone, ME—macular edema, RVO—retinal vein occlusion, SML—subthreshold micropulse laser, VA—visual acuity, VEGF—vascular endothelial growth factor.

4. Discussion

ME significantly reduces visual acuity independently of its cause. Long-standing ME is associated with irreversible visual impairment; thus, the management of this condition should not be delayed.

The resolution of DME is accompanied by macular atrophy due to permanent damage to the photoreceptors, and CST is not a reliable indicator of visual acuity, neither as a prognostic nor as a predictive factor of outcomes [91]. This highlights the importance of evaluating visual acuity as a functional outcome in studies evaluating the effects of ME treatment. Most of the studies reviewed evaluated both central retinal thickness and BCVA, determining its relevance.

Almost all studies comparing laser treatment with other methods of treatment noted that LP has not been the first-line treatment for DME and ME secondary to RVO for some time, as it has been replaced by more effective intravitreal anti-VEGF injections [27–29,77,78].

Although a lower incidence of complications was reported with SML treatment compared with conventional laser treatment, SML treatment has not shown superior effectiveness [31–34]. However, the use of a combined treatment may be an effective and safe alternative for ME treatment and may reduce the number of intravitreal anti-VEGF injections required [34,35].

Although some studies have reported superior efficacy of certain anti-VEGFs over others, the agents reported as superior vary. It is accepted that anti-VEGFs are typically chosen on the basis of baseline VA, drug price, and availability. The new generation of anti-VEGF-A inhibitors, including brolucizumab, abicipar pegol, and conbercept, are believed to be superior to the anti-VEGFs currently used in ME treatment because of their longer intravitreal half-life, higher potency, biochemical properties, and the reduced number of intravitreal injections required per unit time. However, extended studies and trials must be completed before the new drugs are approved [11].

Despite the overall efficacy of anti-VEGFs, many patients do not respond to them. It was reported that only 33–45% of DME patients on anti-VEGF agents showed three lines or more of visual improvement [28]. Forty percent of patients failed to achieve significant visual gains despite 6 months of intensive anti-VEGF therapy. ME persisted in 32% to 66% of eyes and usually affected visual acuity significantly [44].

Despite this, steroids are typically a second choice for both DME and ME due to RVO and are reserved for those who do not respond to anti-VEGF treatment. However, increasing evidence suggests an association between superior functional (increased BCVA) and anatomical (reduced CMT) outcomes and beginning steroid treatment earlier [52,61,63–65]. Although steroids are associated with increased IOP and cataract formation [80], this is not an inevitable outcome for all of the patients treated with steroids, as studies reported these side effects in less than half of patients. In addition, side effects could be caused not only by steroids but also by the preservatives used in their preparation [44]. Most of the studies reported a significant positive effect of intravitreal steroids in the treatment of ME, thus highlighting its advantage. The intravitreal FA implant is superior to the DEX implant because of its longer effect (up to 36 months); however, it is usually used to treat DME in patients who previously received a course of corticosteroids and did not experience a significant increase in eye pressure [11]. Furthermore, intravitreal FA was approved for DME, but it has not yet been approved for ME due to RVO. We did not identify any studies that compared DEX and FA in terms of effectiveness.

It would appear that, as of yet, a consensus on ME treatment has not been reached, particularly in cases that are resistant to standard treatment. We assume that artificial intelligence (AI) may be beneficial in addressing this issue. It was previously reported that AI was able to accurately predict posttreatment central foveal thickness and BCVA after anti-VEGF injections in DME patients; thus, it can be used to prospectively assess the efficacy of anti-VEGF therapy in DME patients [91]. The data regarding AI properties and possibilities in ME diagnosis and treatment prognosis are increasing [92]. Optical coherence tomography (OCT) is an indispensable tool for the application of AI as well as for determining the need for treatment and evaluating its effectiveness in patients with ME [93]. Until AI is widely and effectively incorporated in clinical practice, established imaging biomarkers may significantly contribute to DME management. Hyperreflective retinal foci (HRF) appear as intraretinal hyperreflective dots on OCT in patients with DME and are reported to be an important imaging marker of retinal inflammation [94]. Kim et al. suggested that patients with an increased number of HRF on OCT should be more frequently followed up for early intervention because they observed that a higher number of HRF on the spectral domain (SD) OCT was associated with early recurrence of DME after steroid implants [94]. It was also reported that the presence of subretinal fluid, the absence of HRF, and the integrity of the inner segment–outer segment layer could be OCT biomarkers for superior functional success [55]. Larger cysts (intraretinal cystoid spaces) are associated with poor visual prognosis, and the size of the cyst is correlated with the extent of macular ischemia [14]. An increased fundus autofluorescence (FAF) signal (hyper-autofluorescence) was associated with declining visual acuity and an increase in the macular thickness on OCT [95]. This highlights the properties of FAF as an additional tool that may help monitor the progression of DME and its response to treatment.

5. Perspectives

New therapies, including anti-VEGF-A inhibitors (brolucizumab and abicipar pegol), are under investigation and may be more effective in ME treatment compared with previous anti-VEGFs [11]. A suprachoroidal TA delivery system in DME patients has been investigated as well, and the preliminary results are promising [96]. Nanotechnology was reported to be safe and beneficial in its ability to ensure TA delivery to the retina using topical drops.

The SML is absorbed by xanthophyll pigment, allowing for treatment close to the fovea [84]. It can promote the absorption of edema, hemorrhage, and exudation, and it can improve the retinal oxygen supply and reduce vascular permeability [86]. This relatively new laser technique is superior to a conventional laser because it does not cause structural damage to the retina. Although SML therapy has not shown superiority when used alone in ME treatment, in most of the reviewed studies, SML therapy was reported to be an effective additional treatment method when combined with intravitreal anti-VEGF injections in the treatment of DME and ME due to RVO. Both methods have some limitations and possible complications; however, when combined, they not only effectively reduce ME and increase VA but also reduce the number of intravitreal injections. Therefore, this combined treatment could lower healthcare costs and the burden on patients by reducing the frequency of clinic visits.

With the emerging era of AI, this technology may soon be beneficial in selecting the most effective and appropriate treatment in patients with ME. Promising results were reported in a recent study performed by Gallardo and colleagues [97]. They used machine learning classifiers to predict low and high anti-VEGF treatment demands for patients with DME, RVO, and neovascular age-related macular degeneration treated according to a treat-and-extend regimen. The authors highlighted the ability to predict the low and high treatment demands in all groups of patients with similar accuracy, along with the capability to predict low demand at the first visit before the first injection. Further research is needed to establish the individual treatment demands for patients and consolidate the properties of AI in clinical practice.

Author Contributions: Conceptualization, A.G., A.M. and R.Z.; methodology, A.M.; validation, A.G. and R.Z.; formal analysis, A.M.; investigation, A.G., A.M. and R.Z.; data curation, A.G.; writing—original draft preparation, A.M.; writing—review and editing, A.G., A.M. and R.Z.; visualization, A.G.; supervision, A.G. All authors have read and agreed to the published version of the manuscript.

Funding: This research received no external funding.

Institutional Review Board Statement: Not applicable.

Informed Consent Statement: Not applicable.

Conflicts of Interest: The authors declare no conflict of interest.

References

1. Claudiu, T.S. Agents for the prevention and treatment of age-related macular degeneration and macular edema: A literature and patent review. *Expert Opin. Ther. Pat.* **2019**, *29*, 761–767.
2. Kitazawa, K.; Sotozono, C.; Kinoshita, S. Incidence and Management of Cystoid Macular Edema after Corneal Transplantation. *Int. J. Ophthalmol.* **2017**, *10*, 1081–1087. [CrossRef]
3. Schaub, F.; Adler, W.; Enders, P.; Koenig, M.C.; Koch, K.R.; Cursiefen, C.; Kirchhof, B.; Heindl, L.M. Preexisting epiretinal membrane is associated with pseudophakic cystoid macular edema. *Graefe Arch. Clin. Exp. Ophthalmol.* **2018**, *256*, 909–917. [CrossRef] [PubMed]
4. Aaronson, A.; Achiron, A.; Tuuminen, R. Clinical Course of Pseudophakic Cystoid Macular Edema Treated with Nepafenac. *J. Clin. Med.* **2020**, *9*, 3034. [CrossRef]
5. Walter, K.; Kauffman, L.; Hess, J. Rate of pseudophakic cystoid macular edema using intraoperative and topical nonsteroidal antiinflammatory drugs alone without steroids. *J. Cataract. Refract. Surg.* **2020**, *46*, 350–354. [CrossRef]
6. Koronis, S.; Stavrakas, P.; Balidis, M.; Kozeis, N.; Tranos, P.G. Update in treatment of uveitic macular edema. *Drug Des. Dev. Ther.* **2019**, *13*, 667–680. [CrossRef]
7. Testi, I.; Rousselot, A.; Agrawal, R.; Pavesio, C. Treatment of Uveitic Macular Edema. In *Complications in Uveitis*; Pichi, F., Neri, P., Eds.; Springer: Cham, Switzerland, 2020.
8. Dick, A.D.; Rosenbaum, J.T.; Al-Dhibi, H.A. Guidance on noncorticosteroid systemic immunomodulatory therapy in noninfectious uveitis: Fundamentals of Care for UveitiS (FOCUS) initiative. *Ophthalmology* **2018**, *125*, 757–773. [CrossRef]
9. Liew, G.; Strong, S.; Bradley, P.; Severn, P.; Moore, A.T.; Webster, A.R.; Mitchell, P.; Kifley, A.; Michaelides, M. Prevalence of cystoid macular oedema, epiretinal membrane and cataract in retinitis pigmentosa. *Br. J. Ophthalmol.* **2018**, *103*, 1163–1166. [CrossRef]
10. Petrou, P.; Chalkiadaki, E.; Errera, M.-H.; Liyanage, S.; Wickham, L.; Papakonstantinou, E.; Karamaounas, A.; Kanakis, M.; Georgalas, I.; Kandarakis, S.; et al. Factors Associated with the Clinical Course of Vitreomacular Traction. *J. Ophthalmol.* **2020**, *2020*, 9457670. [CrossRef]
11. Sacconi, R.; Giuffrè, C.; Corbelli, E.; Borrelli, E.; Querques, G.; Bandello, F. Emerging therapies in the management of macular edema: A review. *F1000Research* **2019**, *8*. [CrossRef]
12. Graham, P.S.; Kaidonis, G.; Abhary, S.; Gillies, M.C.; Daniell, M.; Essex, R.W.; Chang, J.H.; Lake, S.R.; Pal, B.; Jenkins, A.J.; et al. Genome-wide association studies for diabetic macular edema and proliferative diabetic retinopathy. *BMC Med. Genet.* **2018**, *19*, 71. [CrossRef]
13. Grassi, M.A.; Tikhomirov, A.; Ramalingam, S.; Below, J.E.; Cox, N.J.; Nicolae, D.L. Genome-wide meta-analysis for severe diabetic retinopathy. *Hum. Mol. Genet.* **2011**, *20*, 2472–2481. [CrossRef]
14. Yalçın, N.G.; Özdek, Ş. The Relationship Between Macular Cyst Formation and Ischemia in Diabetic Macular Edema. *Turk. J. Ophthalmol.* **2019**, *49*, 194–200. [CrossRef]
15. Spooner, K.; Hong, T.; Fraser-Bell, S.; Chang, A. Current Outcomes of Anti-VEGF Therapy in the Treatment of Macular Edema Secondary to Central Retinal Vein Occlusions: A Systematic Review and Meta-Analysis. *Ophthalmologica* **2019**, *242*, 163–177. [CrossRef]
16. Hykin, P.; Prevost, A.T.; Vasconcelos, J.C.; Murphy, C.; Kelly, J.; Ramu, J.; Hounsome, B.; Yang, Y.; Harding, S.P.; Lotery, A.; et al. Clinical Effectiveness of Intravitreal Therapy with Ranibizumab vs Afliber-cept vs Bevacizumab for Macular Edema Secondary to Central Retinal Vein Occlusion: A Randomized Clinical Trial. *JAMA Ophthalmol.* **2019**, *137*, 1256–1264. [CrossRef]

17. Kim, Y.C.; Shin, J.P.; Pak, K.Y.; Kim, H.W.; Sagong, M.; Lee, S.J.; Chung, I.Y.; Park, S.W.; Lee, J.E. Two-year outcomes of the treat-and-extend regimen using aflibercept for treating diabetic macular oedema. *Sci. Rep.* **2020**, *10*, 22030. [CrossRef]
18. Elsebaey, A.E.; Ibrahim, A.M.; Elshaarawy, E.A. Treat-and-extend vs pro re nata regimens of aflibercept in diabetic macular edema. *Menoufia Med. J.* **2020**, *33*, 1144–1149.
19. Ming, S.; Xie, K.; Yang, M.; He, H.; Li, Y.; Lei, B. Comparison of intravitreal dexamethasone implant and anti-VEGF drugs in the treatment of retinal vein occlusion-induced oedema: A meta-analysis and systematic review. *BMJ Open* **2020**, *10*, e032128. [CrossRef]
20. Fonollosa, A.; Llorenç, V.; Artaraz, J.; Jimenez, B.; Ruiz-Arruza, I.; Agirrebengoa, K.; Cordero-Coma, M.; Costales-Mier, F.; Adan, A. Safety and efficacy of intravitreal dexamethasone implants in the management of macular edema secondary to infectious uveitis. *Retina* **2016**, *36*, 1778–1785. [CrossRef]
21. Kim, E.J.; Lin, W.V.; Rodriguez, S.M.; Chen, A.; Loya, A. Treatment of Diabetic Macular Edema. *Curr. Diabetes Rep.* **2019**, *19*, 68. [CrossRef] [PubMed]
22. Romero-Aroca, P. Is Laser Photocoagulation Treatment Currently Useful in Diabetic Macular Edema? *Med. Hypothesis Discov. Innov. Ophthalmol. J.* **2015**, *4*, 5–8.
23. Schmidt-Erfurth, U.; Garcia-Arumi, J.; Bandello, F.; Berg, K.; Chakravarthy, U.; Gerendas, B.S.; Jonas, J.; Larsen, M.; Tadayoni, R.; Loewenstein, A. Guidelines for the Management of Diabetic Macular Edema by the European Society of Retina Specialists (EURETINA). *Ophthalmologica* **2017**, *237*, 185–222. [CrossRef] [PubMed]
24. Karti, O.; Ipek, S.C.; Saatci, A.O. Multimodal Imaging Characteristics of a Large Retinal Capillary Macroaneurism in an Eye with Severe Diabetic Macular Edema: A Case Presentation and Literature Review. *Med. Hypothesis Discov. Innov. Ophthalmol.* **2020**, *9*, 33–37.
25. Castro, F.D.; Matsui, S.R.; Bianchi, G.J.; de Dios-Cuadras, U.; Sahel, J.; Graue Wiechers, F.; Dupas, B.; Paques, M. Indocyanine green angiography for identifying telangiectatic capillaries in diabetic macular oedema. *Br. J. Ophthalmol.* **2020**, *104*, 509–513. [CrossRef]
26. Paques, M.; Philippakis, E.; Bonnet, C.; Falah, S.; Ayello-Scheer, S.; Zwillinger, S.; Girmens, J.-F.; Dupas, B. Indocyanine-green-guided targeted laser photocoagulation of capillary macroaneurysms in macular oedema: A pilot study. *Br. J. Ophthalmol.* **2016**, *101*, 170–174. [CrossRef]
27. Li, X.; Dai, H.; Li, X.; Han, M.; Li, J.; Suhner, A.; Lin, R.; Wolf, S. Efficacy and safety of ranibizumab 0.5 mg in Chinese patients with visual impairment due to diabetic macular edema: Results from the 12-month REFINE study. *Graefe Arch. Clin. Exp. Ophthalmol.* **2019**, *257*, 529–541. [CrossRef]
28. Furino, C.; Boscia, F.; Reibaldi, M.; Alessio, G. Intravitreal Therapy for Diabetic Macular Edema: An Update. *J. Ophthalmol.* **2021**, *2021*, 1–23. [CrossRef]
29. Singh, R.P.; Silva, F.Q.; Gibson, A.; Thompson, D.; Vitti, R.; Berliner, A.J.; Saroj, N. Difference in Treatment Effect Between Intravitreal Aflibercept Injection and Laser by Baseline Factors in Diabetic Macular Edema. *Ophthalmic Surg. Lasers Imaging Retin.* **2019**, *50*, 167–173. [CrossRef]
30. Midena, E.; Micera, A.; Frizziero, L.; Pilotto, E.; Esposito, G.; Bini, S. Sub-threshold micropulse laser treatment reduces inflammatory biomarkers in aqueous humour of diabetic patients with macular edema. *Sci. Rep.* **2019**, *9*, 10034. [CrossRef]
31. Vujosevic, S.; Toma, C.; Villani, E.; Brambilla, M.; Torti, E.; Leporati, F.; Muraca, A.; Nucci, P.; De Cilla, S. Subthreshold Micropulse Laser in Diabetic Macular Edema: 1-Year Improvement in OCT/OCT-Angiography Biomarkers. *Transl. Vis. Sci. Technol.* **2020**, *9*, 31. [CrossRef]
32. Al-Barki, A.; Al-Hijji, L.; High, R.; Schatz, P.; Do, D.; Nguyen, Q.D.; Luttrull, J.K.; Kozak, I. Comparison of short-pulse subthreshold (532 nm) and infrared micropulse (810 nm) macular laser for diabetic macular edema. *Sci. Rep.* **2021**, *11*, 14. [CrossRef] [PubMed]
33. Gawęcki, M. Subthreshold Diode Micropulse Laser Combined with Intravitreal Therapy for Macular Edema—A Systematized Review and Critical Approach. *J. Clin. Med.* **2021**, *10*, 1394. [CrossRef] [PubMed]
34. Altınel, M.G.; Acikalin, B.; Alis, M.G.; Demir, G.; Mutibayraktaroglu, K.M.; Totuk, O.M.G.; Ardagil, A. Comparison of the efficacy and safety of anti-VEGF monotherapy versus anti-VEGF therapy combined with subthreshold micropulse laser therapy for diabetic macular edema. *Lasers Med. Sci.* **2021**, *36*, 1545–1553. [CrossRef] [PubMed]
35. Furashova, O.; Strassburger, P.; Becker, K.; Engelmann, K. Efficacy of combining intravitreal injections of ranibizumab with micro-pulse diode laser versus intravitreal injections of ranibizumab alone in diabetic macular edema (ReCaLL): A single center, randomised, controlled, non-inferiority clinical trial. *BMC Ophthalmol.* **2020**, *20*, 308. [CrossRef]
36. Valera-Cornejo, D.A.; García-Roa, M.; Quiroz-Mendoza, J.; Arias-Gómez, A.; Ramírez-Neria, P.; Villalpando-Gómez, Y.; Romero-Morales, V.; García-Franco, R. Micropulse laser in patients with refractory and treatment-naïve center-involved diabetic macular edema: Short terms visual and anatomic outcomes. *Ther. Adv. Ophthalmol.* **2021**, *13*, 2515841420979112. [CrossRef]
37. Passos, R.M.; Malerbi, F.K.; Rocha, M.; Maia, M.; Farah, M.E. Real-life outcomes of subthreshold laser therapy for diabetic macular edema. *Int. J. Retin. Vitr.* **2021**, *7*, 4. [CrossRef]
38. Wells, J.A.; Glassman, A.R.; Ayala, A.R.; Jampol, L.M.; Bressler, N.M.; Bressler, S.B.; Brucker, A.J.; Ferris, F.L.; Hampton, G.R.; Jhaveri, C.; et al. Aflibercept, Bevacizumab, or Ranibizumab for Diabetic Macular Edema: Two-Year Results from a Comparative Effectiveness Randomized Clinical Trial. *Ophthalmology* **2016**, *123*, 1351–1359. [CrossRef]

39. Bressler, N.M.; Beaulieu, W.T.; Glassman, A.R.; Blinder, K.J.; Bressler, S.B.; Jampol, L.M.; Melia, M.; Wells, J.A. Persistent Macular Thickening Following Intravitreous Aflibercept, Bevacizumab, or Ranibizumab for Central-Involved Diabetic Macular Edema With Vision Impairment: A Secondary Analysis of a Randomized Clinical Trial. *JAMA Ophthalmol.* **2018**, *136*, 257–269. [CrossRef]
40. Haritoglou, C.; Maier, M.; Neubauer, A.S.; Augustin, A.J. Current concepts of pharmacotherapy of diabetic macular edema. *Expert Opin. Pharmacother.* **2020**, *21*, 467–475. [CrossRef]
41. Zhou, Q.; Guo, C.; You, A.; Wang, D.; Wang, W.; Zhang, X. One-year outcomes of novel VEGF decoy receptor therapy with intravitreal conbercept in diabetic retinopathy-induced macular edema. *Mol. Vis.* **2019**, *25*, 636–644.
42. Liu, W.-S.; Li, Y.-J. Comparison of conbercept and ranibizumab for the treatment efficacy of diabetic macular edema: A Meta-analysis and systematic review. *Int. J. Ophthalmol.* **2019**, *12*, 1479–1486. [CrossRef]
43. Sun, X.; Zhang, J.; Tian, J.; Chen, S.; Zeng, F.; Yuan, G. Comparison of the Efficacy and Safety of Intravitreal Conbercept with Intravitreal Ranibizumab for Treatment of Diabetic Macular Edema: A Meta-Analysis. *J. Ophthalmol.* **2020**, 5809081. [CrossRef]
44. Hong, I.H.; Choi, W.; Han, J.R. The effects of intravitreal triamcinolone acetonide in diabetic macular edema refractory to anti-VEGF treatment. *Jpn. J. Ophthalmol.* **2020**, *64*, 196–202. [CrossRef]
45. Fung, A.T.; Tran, T.; Lim, L.L.; Samarawickrama, C.; Arnold, J.; Gillies, M.; Catt, C.; Mitchell, L.; Symons, A.; Buttery, R.; et al. Local delivery of corticosteroids in clinical ophthalmology: A review. *Clin. Exp. Ophthalmol.* **2020**, *48*, 366–401. [CrossRef]
46. Mason, R.H.; Ballios, B.G.; Yan, P. Noninfectious endophthalmitis following intravitreal triamcinolone acetonide: Clinical case and literature review. *Can. J. Ophthalmol.* **2020**, *55*, 471–479. [CrossRef]
47. Lang, Y.; Zemel, E.; Miller, B.; Perlman, I. Retinal toxicity of intravitreal kenalog in albino rabbits. *Retina* **2007**, *27*, 778–788. [CrossRef]
48. Schulze-Döbold, C.; Weber, M. Loss of visual function after repeated intravitreal injections of triamcinolone acetonide in refractory uveitic macular oedema. *Int. Ophthalmol.* **2009**, *29*, 427–429. [CrossRef]
49. Arndt, C.; Meunier, I.; Rebollo, O.; Martinenq, C.; Hamel, C.; Hattenbach, L.-O. Electrophysiological Retinal Pigment Epithelium Changes Observed with Indocyanine Green, Trypan Blue and Triamcinolone. *Ophthalmic Res.* **2010**, *44*, 17–23. [CrossRef]
50. Kodjikian, L.; Bellocq, D.; Bandello, F.; Loewenstein, A.; Chakravarthy, U.; Koh, A.; Augustin, A.; De Smet, M.D.; Chhablani, J.; Tufail, A.; et al. First-line treatment algorithm and guidelines in center-involving diabetic macular edema. *Eur. J. Ophthalmol.* **2018**, *29*, 573–584. [CrossRef]
51. Augustin, A.J.; Feltgen, N.; Haritoglou, C.; Hoerauf, H.; Maier, M.M.; Mardin, C.Y.; Schargus, M. Klinische Entscheidungsfindung bei der Behandlung des diabetischen Makulaödems mit DEX-Implantat: Ein Konsenspapier. *Klin. Monbl. Augenheilkd.* **2019**, *238*, 73–84. [CrossRef]
52. Castro-Navarro, V.; Cervera-Taulet, E.; Navarro-Palop, C.; Monferrer-Adsuara, C.; Hernández-Bel, L.; Montero-Hernández, J. Intravitreal dexamethasone implant Ozurdex® in naïve and refractory patients with different subtypes of diabetic macular edema. *BMC Ophthalmol.* **2019**, *19*, 15. [CrossRef]
53. Medina-Baena, M.; Cejudo-Corbalán, O.; García-Pulido, J.I.; Huertos-Carrillo, M.J.; Girela-López, E. Intravitreal dexamethasone implant in naïve and previously treated patients with diabetic macular edema: A retrospective study. *Int. J. Ophthalmol.* **2020**, *13*, 1597–1605. [CrossRef]
54. Iglicki, M.; Busch, C.; Zur, D.; Huertos-Carrillo, M.J.; Girela-López, E. Dexamethasone implant for diabetic macular edema in naive compared with refractory eyes: The international retina group real-life 24-month multicenter study. The IRGREL-DEX study. *Retina* **2019**, *39*, 44–51. [CrossRef]
55. Altun, A.; Hacimustafaoglu, A.M. Effect of Dexamethasone Implant on Subfoveal Choroidal Thickness in Early Period in Vitrectomized Eyes with Diabetic Macular Edema. *J. Ophthalmol.* **2021**, *2021*, 8840689. [CrossRef]
56. Augustin, A.J.; Bopp, S.; Fechner, M.; Holz, F.; Sandner, D.; Winkgen, A.M.; Khoramnia, R.; Neuhann, T.; Warscher, M.; Spitzer, M.; et al. Three-year results from the Retro-IDEAL study: Real-world data from diabetic macular edema (DME) patients treated with ILUVIEN® (0.19 mg fluocinolone acetonide implant). *Eur. J. Ophthalmol.* **2020**, *30*, 382–391. [CrossRef]
57. Holden, S.E.; Kapik, B.; Beiderbeck, A.B.; Currie, C.J. Comparison of data characterizing the clinical effectiveness of the fluocinolone intravitreal implant (ILUVIEN) in patients with diabetic macular edema from the real world, non-interventional ICE-UK study and the FAME randomized controlled trials. *Curr. Med. Res. Opin.* **2019**, *35*, 1165–1176. [CrossRef]
58. Chakravarthy, U.; Taylor, S.R.; Koch, F.H.J.; De Sousa, J.P.C.; Bailey, C. Changes in intraocular pressure after intravitreal fluocinolone acetonide (ILUVIEN): Real-world experience in three European countries. *Br. J. Ophthalmol.* **2018**, *103*, 1072–1077. [CrossRef]
59. Panos, G.D.; Arruti, N.; Patra, S.; Panos, G.D.; Arruti, N.; Patra, S. The long-term efficacy and safety of fluocinolone acetonide intravitreal implant 190 µg (ILUVIEN®) in diabetic macular oedema in a multi-ethnic inner-city population. *Eur. J. Ophthalmol.* **2021**, *31*, 620–629. [CrossRef]
60. Coelho, J.; Malheiro, L.; Beirão, J.M.; Meireles, A.; Pessoa, B. Real-world retrospective comparison of 0.19 mg fluocinolone acetonide and 0.7 mg dexamethasone intravitreal implants for the treatment of diabetic macular edema in vitrectomized eyes. *Clin. Ophthalmol.* **2019**, *13*, 1751–1759. [CrossRef]
61. Gonzalez, V.H.; Campbell, J.; Holekamp, N.M.; Kiss, S.; Loewenstein, A.; Augustin, A.; Ma, J.; Ho, A.; Patel, V.; Whitcup, S.; et al. Early and long-term responses to anti-vascular endothelial growth factor therapy in diabetic macular edema: Analysis of protocol I data. *Am. J. Ophthalmol.* **2016**, *172*, 72–79. [CrossRef]

62. Baker, C.W.; Glassman, A.R.; Beaulieu, W.T.; Antoszyk, A.N.; Browning, D.J.; Chalam, K.V.; Grover, S.; Jampol, L.M.; Jhaveri, C.D.; Melia, M.; et al. Effect of initial management with aflibercept vs laser photocoagulation vs observation on vision loss among patients with diabetic macular edema involving the center of the macular and good visual acuity: A randomized clinical trial. *JAMA* **2019**, *321*, 1880–1894. [CrossRef] [PubMed]
63. Martínez, A.H.; Delgado, E.P.; Silva, G.S.; Mateos, L.C.; Pascual, J.L.; Villa, J.L.; Vicente, P.G.; Almeida-González, C.-V. Early versus late switch: How long should we extend the anti-vascular endothelial growth factor therapy in unresponsive diabetic macular edema patients? *Eur. J. Ophthalmol.* **2019**, *30*, 1091–1098. [CrossRef] [PubMed]
64. Demir, G.; Ozkaya, A.; Yuksel, E.; Erdogan, G.; Tunc, U.; Ocal, M.C.; Göker, Y. Early and Late Switch from Ranibizumab to an Intravitreal Dexamethasone Implant in Patients with Diabetic Macular Edema in the Event of a Poor Anatomical Response. *Clin. Drug Investig.* **2019**, *40*, 119–128. [CrossRef] [PubMed]
65. Ruiz-Medrano, J.; Rodríguez-Leor, R.; Almazán, E.; Lugo, F.; Casado-Lopez, E.; Arias, L.; Ruiz-Moreno, J.M. Results of dexamethasone intravitreal implant (Ozurdex) in diabetic macular edema patients: Early versus late switch. *Eur. J. Ophthalmol.* **2020**, *31*, 1135–1145. [CrossRef] [PubMed]
66. Panozzo, G.A.; Gusson, E.; Panozzo, G.; Dalla Mura, G. Dexamethasone intravitreal implant at the time of cataract surgery in eyes with diabetic macular edema. *Eur. J. Ophthalmol.* **2017**, *27*, 433–437. [CrossRef]
67. Furino, C.; Boscia, F.; Niro, A.; Giancipoli, E.; Grassi, M.O.; Ricci, G.D.; Blasetti, F.; Reibaldi, M.; Alessio, G. Combined Phacoemulsification and Intravitreal Dexamethasone Implant (Ozurdex®) in Diabetic Patients with Coexisting Cataract and Diabetic Macular Edema. *J. Ophthalmol.* **2017**, *2017*, 4896036. [CrossRef] [PubMed]
68. Calvo, P.; Ferreras, A.; Al Adel, F.; Dangboon, W.; Brent, M.H. Effect of an intravitreal dexamethasone implant on diabetic macular edema after cataract surgery. *Retina* **2018**, *38*, 490–496. [CrossRef]
69. Furino, C.; Boscia, F.; Niro, A.; D'Addario, M.; Grassi, M.O.; Saglimbene, V.; Reibaldi, M.; Alessio, G. Diabetic macular edema and cataract surgery: Phacoemulsification Combined with Dexamethasone Intravitreal Implant Compared with Standard Phacoemulsification. *Retina* **2021**, *41*, 1102–1109. [CrossRef]
70. Mansour, A.M.; Stewart, M.W.; Farah, M.E.; Mansour, H.A.; Chhablani, J. Ziv-aflibercept: A cost-effective, off-label, highly potent antagonist of vascular endothelial growth factor. *Acta Ophthalmol.* **2019**, *98*. [CrossRef]
71. De Andrade, G.C.; Dias, J.R.D.O.; Maia, A.; Farah, M.E.; Meyer, C.H.; Rodrigues, E.B. Intravitreal Ziv-Aflibercept for Diabetic Macular Edema: 48-Week Outcomes. *Ophthalmic Surg. Lasers Imaging Retin.* **2018**, *49*, 245–250. [CrossRef]
72. Sahni, J.; Patel, S.S.; Dugel, P.U.; Khanani, A.; Jhaveri, C.; Wykoff, C.; Hershberger, V.; Pauly-Evers, M.; Sadikhov, S.; Szczesny, P.; et al. Simultaneous Inhibition of Angiopoietin-2 and Vascular Endothelial Growth Factor-A with Faricimab in Diabetic Macular Edema: BOULEVARD Phase 2 Randomized Trial. *Ophthalmology* **2019**, *126*, 1155–1170. [CrossRef]
73. Yanet, G.; Moreno, C.; Rivera, I.; Altamirano, G.; Padilla, E.; Heald, A.; Moreno, G. Lutein Supplementation for Diabetic Macular Edema. *Food Sci. Nutr. Res.* **2019**, *2*, 1–3.
74. Zhang, Y.; Duan, J.; Chang, T.; Li, X.; Wang, M.; Zhang, M. Comparative efficacy of intravitreal pharmacotherapy for macular edema secondary to retinal vein occlusion: A protocol for the systematic review and network meta-analysis. *Medicine* **2020**, *99*, e22267. [CrossRef]
75. Xia, J.-P.; Wang, S.; Zhang, J.-S. The anti-inflammatory and anti-oxidative effects of conbercept in treatment of macular edema secondary to retinal vein occlusion. *Biochem. Biophys. Res. Commun.* **2018**, *508*, 1264–1270. [CrossRef]
76. Hayreh, S.S. Photocoagulation for retinal vein occlusion. *Prog. Retin. Eye Res.* **2021**, 100964. [CrossRef]
77. Qian, T.; Zhao, M.; Xu, X.; Qian, T. Comparison between anti-VEGF therapy and corticosteroid or laser therapy for macular oedema secondary to retinal vein occlusion: A meta-analysis. *J. Clin. Pharm. Ther.* **2017**, *42*, 519–529. [CrossRef]
78. Ogura, Y.; Kondo, M.; Kadonosono, K.; Shimura, M.; Kamei, M.; Tsujikawa, A. Current practice in the management of branch retinal vein occlusion in Japan: Survey results of retina specialists in Japan. *Jpn. J. Ophthalmol.* **2019**, *63*, 365–373. [CrossRef]
79. Feng, X.-X.; Li, C.; Shao, W.-W.; Yuan, Y.-G.; Qian, X.-B.; Zheng, Q.-S.; Li, Y.-J.; Gao, Q.-Y. Intravitreal anti-VEGF agents, oral glucocorticoids, and laser photocoagulation combination therapy for macular edema secondary to retinal vein occlusion: Preliminary report. *Int. J. Ophthalmol.* **2018**, *11*, 429–437. [CrossRef]
80. Costa, J.V.; Moura-Coelho, N.; Abreu, A.C.; Neves, P.; Ornelas, M.; Furtado, M.J. Macular edema secondary to retinal vein occlusion in a real-life setting: A multicenter, nationwide, 3-year follow-up study. *Graefe Arch. Clin. Exp.* **2021**, *259*, 343–350. [CrossRef]
81. Liu, W.; Li, Y.; Cao, R.; Bai, Z.; Liu, W. A systematic review and meta-analysis to compare the efficacy of conbercept with ranibizumab in patients with macular edema secondary to retinal vein occlusion. *Medicine* **2020**, *99*, e20222. [CrossRef]
82. Arrigo, A.; Crepaldi, A.; Viganò, C.; Aragona, E.; Lattanzio, R.; Scalia, G.; Resti, A.G.; Calcagno, F.; Pina, A.; Rashid, H.F.; et al. Real-Life Management of Central and Branch Retinal Vein Occlusion: A Seven-Year Follow-Up Study. *Thromb. Haemost.* **2021**, *121*, 1361–1366. [CrossRef] [PubMed]
83. Buyru, Ö.Y.; Akkaya, S.; Aksoy, S.; Şimşek, M.H. Comparison of ranibizumab and subthreshold micropulse laser in treatment of macular edema secondary to branch retinal vein occlusion. *Eur. J. Ophthalmol.* **2018**, *28*, 690–696. [CrossRef] [PubMed]
84. Eng, V.A.; Leng, T. Subthreshold laser therapy for macular oedema from branch retinal vein occlusion: Focused review. *Br. J. Ophthalmol.* **2020**. [CrossRef] [PubMed]

85. Terashima, H.; Hasebe, H.; Okamoto, F.; Matsuoka, N.; Sato, Y.; Fukuchi, T. Combination therapy of intravitreal ranibizumab and subthreshold micropulse photocoagulation for macular edema secondary to branch retinal vein occlusion: 6-month result. *Retina* **2019**, *39*, 1377–1384. [CrossRef]
86. Chen, G.; Chen, P.; Chen, X.; Wang, J.; Peng, X. The laser combined with intravitreal injection of ranibizumab for treatment of macular edema secondary to branch retinal vein occlusion: A protocol for systematic review and meta-analysis. *Medicine* **2021**, *100*, e23675. [CrossRef]
87. Navarro-Partida, J.; Altamirano-Vallejo, J.C.; Lopez-Naranjo, E.J.; la Rosa, A.G.-D.; Manzano-Ramírez, A.; Apatiga-Castro, L.M.; Armendáriz-Borunda, J.; Santos, A. Topical Triamcinolone Acetonide-Loaded Liposomes as Primary Therapy for Macular Edema Secondary to Branch Retinal Vein Occlusion: A Pilot Study. *J. Ocul. Pharmacol. Ther.* **2020**, *36*, 393–403. [CrossRef]
88. Cheng, T.; Li, J.; Cheng, Y.; Zhang, X.; Qu, Y. Triamcinolone acetonide-chitosan coated liposomes efficiently treated retinal edema as eye drops. *Exp. Eye Res.* **2019**, *188*, 107805. [CrossRef]
89. Kida, T.; Flammer, J.; Konieczka, K.; Ikeda, T. Retinal venous pressure is decreased after anti-VEGF therapy in patients with retinal vein occlusion-related macular edema. *Graefe Arch. Clin. Exp. Ophthalmol.* **2021**, *259*, 1853–1858. [CrossRef]
90. Rothman, A.L.; Thomas, A.S.; Khan, K.; Fekrat, S. Central retinal vein occlusion in young individuals. *Retina* **2019**, *39*, 1917–1924. [CrossRef]
91. Markan, A.; Agarwal, A.; Arora, A.; Bazgain, K.; Rana, V.; Gupta, V. Novel imaging biomarkers in diabetic retinopathy and diabetic macular edema. *Ther. Adv. Ophthalmol.* **2020**, *12*. [CrossRef]
92. Liu, B.; Zhang, B.; Hu, Y.; Cao, D.; Yang, D.; Wu, Q.; Hu, Y.; Yang, J.; Peng, Q.; Huang, M.; et al. Automatic prediction of treatment outcomes in patients with diabetic macular edema using ensemble machine learning. *Ann. Transl. Med.* **2021**, *9*, 43. [CrossRef]
93. Hecht, I.; Bar, A.; Rokach, L.; Achiron, R.; Munk, M.; Huf, W.; Burgansky-Eliash, Z.; Achiron, A. Optical coherence tomography biomarkers to distinguish diabetic macular edema from pseudophakic cystoid macular edema using machine learning algorithms. *Retina* **2019**, *39*, 2283–2291. [CrossRef]
94. Kim, K.T.; Kim, D.Y.; Chae, J.B. Association between Hyperreflective Foci on Spectral-Domain Optical Coherence Tomography and Early Recurrence of Diabetic Macular Edema after Intravitreal Dexamethasone Implantation. *J. Ophthalmol.* **2019**, *2019*, 3459164. [CrossRef]
95. Özmen, S.; Ağca, S.; Doğan, E.; Aksoy, N.; Çakır, B.; Sonalcan, V.; Alagöz, G. Evaluation of fundus autofluorescence imaging of diabetic patients without retinopathy. *Arq. Bras. Oftalmol.* **2019**, *82*, 412–416. [CrossRef]
96. Clearside Biomedical, Inc. Suprachoroidal CLS-TA with Intravitreal Aflibercept versus Aflibercept alone in Subject with Diabetic Macular Edema (TYBEE). Available online: https://clinicaltrials.gov/ct2/show/NCT03126786 (accessed on 27 June 2021).
97. Gallardo, M.; Munk, M.R.; Kurmann, T.; De Zanet, S.; Mosinska, A.; Karagoz, I.K.; Zinkernagel, M.S.; Wolf, S.; Sznitman, R. Machine Learning Can Predict Anti-VEGF Treatment Demand in a Treat-and-Extend Regimen for Patients with Neovascular AMD, DME, and RVO Associated Macular Edema. *Ophthalmol. Retina* **2021**, *5*, 604–624. [CrossRef]

Journal of
Clinical Medicine

Review

Update on the Management of Uveitic Macular Edema

Slawomir Jan Teper

Clinical Department of Ophthalmology, Faculty of Medical Sciences in Zabrze, Medical University of Silesia, 40-760 Katowice, Poland; slawomir.teper@sum.edu.pl

Abstract: Uveitic macular edema (ME) is a frequent complication in 8.3% of uveitis patients and is a leading cause of serious visual impairment in about 40% of cases. Despite the numerous available drugs for its treatment, at least a third of patients fail to achieve satisfactory improvement in visual acuity. First-line drugs are steroids administered by various routes, but drug intolerance or ineffectiveness occur frequently, requiring the addition of other groups of therapeutic drugs. Immunomodulatory and biological drugs can have positive effects on inflammation and often on the accompanying ME, but most uveitic randomized clinical trials to date have not aimed to reduce ME; hence, there is no clear scientific evidence of their effectiveness in this regard. Before starting therapy to reduce general or local immunity, infectious causes of inflammation should be ruled out. This paper discusses local and systemic drugs, including steroids, biological drugs, immunomodulators, VEGF inhibitors, and anti-infection medication.

Keywords: macular edema; uveitis; uveitic complications; non-steroidal anti-inflammatory drugs; steroids; biologic treatment

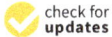

Citation: Teper, S.J. Update on the Management of Uveitic Macular Edema. *J. Clin. Med.* **2021**, *10*, 4133. https://doi.org/10.3390/jcm10184133

Academic Editor: Gawęcki Maciej

Received: 15 August 2021
Accepted: 11 September 2021
Published: 14 September 2021

Publisher's Note: MDPI stays neutral with regard to jurisdictional claims in published maps and institutional affiliations.

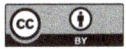

Copyright: © 2021 by the author. Licensee MDPI, Basel, Switzerland. This article is an open access article distributed under the terms and conditions of the Creative Commons Attribution (CC BY) license (https://creativecommons.org/licenses/by/4.0/).

1. Introduction

Uveitis is a common cause of blindness, especially at working age and in low- or middle-income countries [1,2]. There are many causes of blindness or significant visual impairment in patients with uveitis, but the most common and important is macular edema (ME), which affects about 40% of patients with 20/60 visual acuity or less, according to [3]. There are many causes of ME, but secondary edema caused by uveitis has perhaps one of the most complex and varied pathomechanisms [4]. ME occurs in 8.3% of non-infectious uveitis patients [4]. It can persist without any sign of concurrent inflammation, but active inflammation can make ME difficult to treat.

Inflammatory ME is a complication of a heterogeneous group of diseases with complex etiologies, which makes multicenter clinical trials for uveitic ME difficult and expensive, and a lack of high-quality evidence-based medical data hinders guideline development. Despite the striking increase in related studies in recent decades, many clinical decisions in uveitis cases are not supported by strong scientific evidence. This paper therefore reviews the available methods of treating ME, together with their advantages and disadvantages, and indicates appropriate therapies for specific clinical situations. Proper uveitis management that considers the etiology in a specific case is sometimes enough to restore normal retinal thickness, but many patients require additional treatment dedicated to ME. Infectious cases, in which an eradication of the infection suffices, are an exception. Thus, this paper proposes treatment for ME following infections, focusing on the treatment of ME itself rather than etiological factors. Acute treatment usually involves the use of steroids via various routes of administration. Long-term treatment, however, should avoid the use of steroid drugs because of their common side effects.

2. Infectious Uveitis
Anti-Infection Agents

ME may be secondary to an infection, and aggressive steroid or intravitreal treatment should not be started until infection has been ruled out. Table 1 lists the most common pathogens involved in ME, together with examples of treatment regimens. Besides the pathogens listed in the table, many other viruses, bacteria, fungi, and parasites can be responsible for ME.

Table 1. Common infectious causes of uveitis and ME (in alphabetical order) along with treatment options.

Pathogen	Examples of Treatment Regimens
Bartonella sp.	Treatment remains controversial. Doxycycline 100 mg bid, alone or in combination with rifampin 300 mg bid; fluoroquinolones; or macrolides + steroids (e.g., Prednisolone 60 mg/day). Treatment should continue for a few weeks [5].
Borrelia sp.	Oral doxycycline 100 mg bid or intravenous ceftriaxone 1 g/day + steroids (e.g., oral prednisolone 1 mg/kg/day) [6].
Herpes sp.	Oral Valacyclovir 1–3 g/day or acyclovir 5 × 800 mg/day + intravitreal foscarnet 2.4 mg/0.1 mL twice weekly [7].
Mycobacterium tuberculosis	Multidrug therapy with four drugs (isoniazid, rifampin, ethambutol, and pyrazinamide) according to the country's health policy [8].
Treponema pallidum (syphilis)	Intravenous aqueous penicillin G 18–24 MU/day every 4 h for 10–14 days + oral or intravenous steroids [9].
Toxocara sp.	Poor visual outcomes are common despite treatment: albendazole + steroids or vitrectomy in severe cases [10].
Toxoplasma sp.	Oral six-week course of clindamycin, pyrimethamine " sulfadiazine, or trimethoprim/sulfamethoxazole + a tapering course of oral prednisolone (1 mg/kg) [11].

3. Non-Infectious Uveitis
3.1. Local Treatment

The advantage of local eye treatment is usually its negligible effect on other organs. The disadvantage is that it treats only one eye, whereas inflammatory ME often affects both eyes. Moreover, obtaining a high drug concentration requires either a frequent use of the drug or an invasive administration route. The emergence of long-acting drugs administered locally has contributed to the increasing popularity of such treatment.

3.1.1. Topical Steroids

Corticosteroids are first-line agents for addressing inflammation in most acute uveitis cases. However, the topical route of administration limits their effectiveness to only mild ME following anterior uveitis. Dexamethasone can be used frequently. Usually, when initiating treatment for acute anterior uveitis, corticosteroids are given every 1 h except during the night. Although application every 15 min can be even more effective, this dosing is only possible for a brief period. As the inflammation subsides over the following days or weeks, the eye drops can be used less frequently, but discontinuation of treatment before at least a few weeks may cause a rapid relapse. In terms of ME, it can be used only in cases of anterior uveitis—usually for patients with rather mild or no ME. No reports have confirmed their efficacy for treating uveitic ME.

3.1.2. Topical Non-Steroidal Anti-Inflammatory Drugs (NSAIDs)

The activity of cyclooxygenases during inflammation promotes the increased production of prostaglandins, which in turn increases vascular permeability and contributes to ME. Although NSAIDs seem to be an excellent treatment choice, pseudophakic ME does not share the same cytokine profile as uveitic ME, and clinical trials have not confirmed the efficacy of topical drugs; hence, they are now used for pseudophakic ME or as a controversial adjunct to corticosteroids for uveitis. Their effectiveness for uveitic ME has not been clearly proven, and their effects are often of borderline statistical significance [12]. Scientific publications have mentioned, for example, bromfenac and nepafenac for this indication [13,14]. Usually, NSAIDs are administered three times daily, but bromfenac seems to be sufficient twice a day for pseudophakic ME [13].

3.1.3. Topical Interferons

Topical interferons are used off-label because there is no topical formulation on the market, but they should be prepared by a pharmacy. In many countries, the availability of INF-α2a (Roferon-A®) or INF-α2b (Intron-A®) is limited, and scientific reports on their topical administration are also limited; consequently, they are rarely prescribed. INF-α and TNF-α have opposite effects in inflammation. Reports have shown the efficacy of topical administration four times a day for both uveitic and diabetic ME [15–17].

3.1.4. Periocular Steroids

Periocular drug administration can be divided into subconjunctival, peribulbar, and retrobulbar injections; injections under the Tenon capsule; and a relatively new route, suprachoroidal injections. In each of these cases, the drugs used for uveitic ME are steroids.

Subconjunctival Steroids

For inflammation in the anterior region of the eye, subconjunctival steroids are often used, but their use for ME is much less frequent and is associated with lower penetration into the posterior region and a relatively short duration of action, especially for dexamethasone.

Frequent (e.g., five times a day) subconjunctival dexamethasone injections increase steroid concentration in the eye, but are inconvenient for the patient and the ophthalmologist, and the efficacy is transitory. Since treatment of ME is necessarily long term, dexamethasone administration is not used for this purpose.

The use of long-acting steroids seems to be the right choice for subconjunctival administration. However, although further studies have been called for, especially for economic reasons, no multicenter randomized studies have compared this option with others [18].

So far, the published results for such treatment are promising—CST reduction occurs in most patients, with accompanying improvement in visual acuity and relapses in only about a quarter of patients six months after an injection [19]. Unfortunately, this route of administration can have side effects, especially in the form of an increase in IOP (25% of participants), with some patients requiring surgical rinsing out of triamcinolone.

Other reported local side effects, such as conjunctival ulceration, necrosis, and infectious scleritis, are rare [20,21].

Subtenon/Peribulbar Steroids

Injections under the Tenon capsule have been performed for over 50 years, and although the first report concerned optic neuritis [22], it was quickly realized that this route was also useful for uveitis [23]. A complication for ophthalmologists performing this procedure is possible perforation of the eyeball, which can be avoided by moving the needle sideways during the injection.

As with the administration of steroids by other routes, an increase in IOP is a common adverse effect depending on the dose and location of the drug [24]. Rearward injections appear to have a lower risk of significantly increasing IOP [25].

Elevated IOP (>21 mm Hg) can be expected in about 15–20% of uveitic patients following triamcinolone injections, and an increase in IOP above 5 mm Hg has been observed in roughly a third of patients [26]. However, some papers have reported ocular hypertension in more than 75% of patients receiving subtenon triamcinolone, with a 23% incidence of glaucoma in the follow-up period [27].

Suprachoroidal Route

The method of delivering medications between the choroid and the sclera was devised to increase the concentration of drugs in the posterior pole of the eye more effectively than administration under the Tenon capsule or into the vitreous. This method is still under investigation, but the results so far are very promising, with a special triamcinolone formula administered in this way being developed. The results of the six-month phase 3 PEACHTREE study showed that the efficacy and safety profile was satisfactory, and this was confirmed by the MAGNOLIA study. Almost half the patients who were treated with suprachoroidally injected triamcinolone acetonide formulation (CLS-TA)—a suspension of triamcinolone acetonide—gained 15 or more ETDRS letters for BCVA versus 16% in the control group ($p < 0.001$), and the mean improvement was 9.6 versus 1.3 letters. The mean reduction in CST from the baseline was 153 μm versus 18 μm ($p < 0.001$), and elevated intraocular pressure occurred in 11.5% and 15.6% of the CLS-TA and control groups, respectively. Cataract AE rates were also similar (7.3% vs. 6.3%, respectively). The control group received sham injections. However, this leaves the basic question unanswered: Would administering triamcinolone periocularly in a different way or directly into the vitreous achieve better results? [28]

3.1.5. Intravitreal Route

A high drug concentration can be obtained by an injection into the vitreous. Currently, intravitreal injections are the most frequently performed invasive ophthalmic procedure in the world due to the introduction of VEGF inhibitors. Although uveitis is not one of the most common indications for their use, they have often proved effective. Uveitis can lead to the development of choroidal neovascularization, so treatment with VEGF inhibitors is the treatment of choice, but anti-VEGF agents are often used successfully for inflammatory ME. Nevertheless, steroids are the primary medications administered intravitreally for uveitis. Unlike previous routes of drug administration, there is a possibility of infectious pathogens entering the vitreous, causing a risk of endophthalmitis. This risk is especially significant in the case of steroids (up to about 0.15–0.5% of injections) [29–31].

Steroids

Currently, some steroids are used intravitreally, differing primarily in their duration of action but sharing common side effects. Although the longest possible duration of action is always crucial for treating ME, treatment should not begin with the longest-acting steroids. The initial use of shorter-acting drugs prevents a surprise increase in IOP and the potential need for a vitrectomy to remove the steroid from the vitreous chamber. Despite the known differences between steroids, specific pharmacokinetics in particular patients have hardly been estimated, and there can be notable differences in the duration of action after using the same drug. Although triamcinolone is assumed to be shorter acting than Ozurdex®, it is impossible to predict the specific duration of action before its first use in a patient.

Triamcinolone acetonide is one of the most common intravitreally injected steroids that is used off-label, and there are many pharmacological triamcinolone products on the market. For many years, it was believed that the benzyl alcohol (preservative) content increased the risk of sterile endophthalmitis, especially in the presence of uveitis. Although this cannot be fully ruled out, studies have also suggested that the triamcinolone crystal size is more important than the preservative composition [32]. Due to limited solubility of triamcinolone, the desired concentration in the vitreous lasts for about three months after a single injection. The most common dose is 4 mg, but 2 mg is also used. Significant improvement in visual acuity has been observed in about 50% of patients. In most cases, repeated injections are needed to avoid ME relapses. Cataract progression relates to the number of injections, and 4–5 administrations almost always result in cataract formation. Increased IOP (in 20–45% of patients) is usually transient and easily managed with IOP-lowering medication.

The remaining drugs in this group are steroid devices, which, by slowly releasing the active substance (dexamethasone or fluocinolone), ensure many months or years of action. Because the implantation of such devices is more difficult than intravitreal injections, comparatively major surgical complications can be expected. In a retrospective analysis of 1241 dexamethasone implantations, 1.69% procedures led to complications, including displacement of the implant by corneal decompensation or hypotony, especially with preexisting risk factors (e.g., in post-PPV eyes) [33].

Ozurdex® (a 700-µg dexamethasone intravitreal implant; AbbVie, Chicago, IL, USA) is a polymer-based, sustained-release corticosteroid formulation implanted into the vitreous, which has the shortest duration of action among the polymer drug group. The HURON study found that the proportion of eyes with a vitreous haze score of 0 at week 8 was 47% with a dexamethasone implant and 12% with a sham ($p < 0.001$)—a benefit that persisted through week 26. However, in terms of ME, a significant decrease in CST was seen at week 8, which did not persist until week 26 [34].

In the POINT six-month trial, periocular triamcinolone acetonide (PTA), intravitreal triamcinolone acetonide (ITA), and an intravitreal dexamethasone implant (IDI) were directly compared with randomization at 1:1:1. The study aimed to measure their influence on ME relative to the proportion of CST at baseline and CST at eight weeks (CST at 8 weeks/CST at BL) assessed with optical coherence tomography (OCT). Reductions of 23%, 39%, and 46% for PTA, ITA, and IDI were observed, respectively; thus, the intravitreal route was superior, but with no difference between drugs. The risk of an IOP of ≥24 mm Hg was higher in the intravitreal treatment groups than in the periocular group (95% CI: 1.83, 0.91–3.65 and 2.52, 1.29–4.91 for ITA and IDI, respectively), with no significant difference between the two intravitreal treatment groups [35].

Ozurdex® insertion must be repeated more often than with Retisert® or Iluvien®, so it is inconvenient to compare adverse events with those for other sustained-release devices. In a retinal vein occlusion (RVO) 24-month trial, cataract progression was observed in almost 40% of patients and an IOP increase in about 35% [36]. Since implantations can lead to vitreous infections, they can increase the risk of endophthalmitis compared to other steroid devices.

Iluvien® (a 0.19 mg fluocinolone acetonide intravitreal implant; Alimera Sciences Ltd., England, UK) continuously releases 0.2 mg/day of fluocinolone to the posterior segment of the eye over a 36-month period. In a 36-month randomized trial, the time to first recurrence of uveitis was substantially longer than for the sham group—657 versus 70.5 days. ME was an additional outcome—more than two times fewer patients had investigator-determined ME in the treatment group than in the sham group (13.0% vs. 27.3%). It is worth noting that this result was not statistically significant ($p = 0.079$) and was mentioned only in the main text of the paper. Adjunctive treatment was received by 95.7% of patients in the sham group and 57.5% in the treated group, but the impact of these additional therapies on ME could not be determined. The lack of statistical significance could have been related to the size of the treated group—only about 60% of people had edema at the baseline, so the sample size was not sufficient for confirming ME. IOP-lowering medications were needed for 42.5% of the treated eyes and 33.3% of the sham group. Glaucoma surgery was needed for 11.9% of the treated eyes and 5.7% of the sham group. Furthermore, 73.8% versus 23.8% of phakic eyes required cataract surgery, respectively, in the treated and sham groups [37].

Retisert® (a 0.59 mg fluocinolone acetonide intravitreal implant; Bausch & Lomb, Rochester, New York, NY, USA) is a sustained-release system designed to deliver corticosteroids inside the eye for up to 30 months. ME was a secondary efficacy outcome in a 36-month historically controlled clinical trial; since there was no control group, reduction of ME areas relative to ME in the fellow eyes were analyzed. Uveitis recurrence was reduced in implanted eyes from 62% (during the one-year preimplantation period) to 4%, 10%, and 20% (during the one-, two-, and three-year postimplantation periods, respectively). At the one- and three-year visits, the CME area was reduced in 86% and 73% of implantation cases compared with 28% and 28% in fellow nonimplanted eyes, respectively. An 80% reduction in systemic medications was needed as an adjunctive therapy during the postimplantation period. However, it was difficult to accurately trace the changes in concomitant treatment and their potential impact on ME from the article text. A greater than 10 mm Hg increase in IOP was noted in 67% of patients after implantation, and 40% of patients required glaucoma surgery. Over 90% of patients required cataract surgery in the fluocinolone implanted eyes during the study (compared to 20% in the fellow phakic eyes) [38].

VEGF Inhibitors

An increasing number of anti-VEGF agents have entered the market. Although a few have been registered for ophthalmology, this registration does not apply to uveitic ME; therefore, treatment, regardless of the choice of drug, is off-label. For patients who are steroid intolerant or phakic, VEGF inhibitors could be the treatment of choice. VEGF is a major vascular permeability factor and is heavily involved in the development of uveitic ME of various origins [39]. Given how frequently VEGF inhibitors are used in ophthalmology, it may come as a surprise that so little scientific evidence has been published for their efficacy in uveitic ME. Unlike steroid preparations, no VEGF inhibitors have such long durations of action. Currently, bevacizumab, ranibizumab, and aflibercept are used for other indications, but it is worth noting that anti-VEGF drugs—particularly brolucizumab–have the potential to cause inflammation, including occlusive retinal vasculitis [40]. No specific anti-VEGF treatment regimen for uveitic ME has been proposed so far. It is not known whether VEGF inhibitors should be used for people with infectious uveitis and ME, in cases where the use of immunosuppressing drugs may be harmful. It is also unclear whether it is necessary to wait for the inflammation to decrease or be eliminated before starting this treatment. Some studies have reported positive effects of anti-VEGF drugs (ranibizumab, bevacizumab, and aflibercept) on uveitic ME; the administration of subsequent injections was usually associated with a relapse or worsening of edema measured by OCT [41–43].

Immunomodulatory Agents

Methotrexate—an antifolate antimetabolite—can be injected into the vitreous to avoid systemic manifestations of adverse effects when inflammation is still active. In a prospective case study with 15 participants who all had intermediate or posterior ME or panuveitis, 400 µg/0.1 mL methotrexate was administered, and it improved ocular inflammation scores. On average, macular thickness decreased from 425 to 275 µm over the six-month period of observation. One third of patients relapsed at a median time of four months, but reinjection was as effective as after first injection. One (pseudophakic) patient developed corneal decompensation—which could be treated with topical folinic acid [44]. Although a larger study was conducted, it provided no detailed data regarding ME [45]. Cataracts are likely to develop less frequently with methotrexate than with steroid drugs, but due to short treatment times and small sample populations, it was impossible to identify the incidence of cataract as an adverse event in those groups.

Intravitreal sirolimus—an mTOR inhibitor—may be effective in some cases of uveitic ME; however, the SAVE-2 trial failed to achieve statistical significance in reducing ME. It may be crucial to select the right patients for sirolimus treatment of ME, since some participants showed significant improvement and others worsened during treatment [46].

3.2. Systemic Treatment

3.2.1. Steroids

Systemic steroids are very effective for treating uveitic CME, but their use is limited due to their numerous systemic side effects. Discontinuation of medication often results in a recurrence of edema, necessitating re-treatment and associated adverse events. It is important to identify a personalized minimal effective dose—usually starting with 0.5–1 mg of prednisone/kg or an equivalent dose of other steroids [47]. The most used medications include oral prednisone and methylprednisolone. Systemic steroids are chosen more frequently for bilateral cases than for unilateral cases. ME is one of the factors contributing to the choice of oral steroids for uveitis, but oral corticosteroids are also one of the major strategies in relapse in uveitis without ME [48]. The side effects of systemic steroids are numerous and usually dose-dependent; therefore, chronic oral use is almost always destructive to the human body, from the skeletal system to the brain [47].

3.2.2. Immunomodulatory Agents

Systemic treatment with immunosuppressive agents can effectively reduce ME associated with active inflammation. However, patients should be made aware that immunomodulating drugs are not panaceas for ocular complications. Evaluating immunosuppressive therapy in uveitis is very challenging. Only 19 randomized clinical trials of immunomodulating drugs for intermediate and posterior uveitis could be found in the medical databases, but these studies did not always present ME data, or the researchers observed positive trends toward reducing macular thickness but without statistical significance [49]. In the absence of relevant data, a retrospective analysis was warranted. This was conducted by the SITE study, which examined the past use of antimetabolites, T-cell inhibitors, alkylating agents, and other immunosuppressives based on the medical records of approximately 9250 uveitis patients at five tertiary centers over 30 years [50]. Of more than 1500 eyes, 52% showed improved visual acuity of at least the equivalent of two lines on an ETDRS chart [51]. Negative prognostic factors—snow banking (not snowballs), posterior synechiae, and hypotony—were also identified. The SITE study aimed to check whether the most-used immunosuppressive drugs led to increased cancer-related or overall mortality. The results suggested that tumor necrosis factor inhibitors could increase mortality, but this was not evident in patients treated with azathioprine, methotrexate, mycophenolate mofetil, ciclosporin, systemic corticosteroids, or dapsone (only cyclophosphamide was an exception among immunomodulatory agents) [52].

3.2.3. Biologic Agents

No completed or ongoing clinical trials have confirmed or contradicted the efficacy of anti-TNF agents for uveitic ME [53]. However, based on some reports, it seems that, in at least some patient groups, subcutaneous TNF-alpha inhibitors may be effective for ME when used at standard doses [54].

3.2.4. Interferons

In a two-pronged study, either interferon beta 44 mg was administered subcutaneously three times weekly or 20 mg MTX was administered subcutaneously once weekly; macular thickness decreased by a mean of 206 μm in the interferon group but increased by 47 μm in the methotrexate group ($p < 0.0001$) [55].

Interferon alpha2a has been used successfully to treat Behçet's disease and other types of uveitis (about 60% efficacy in reducing inflammation). It can be even more effective for treating uveitic ME—one study reported control of ME in more than 80% of patients receiving subcutaneous interferon alpha2a [56]. Major but rare side effects (in about 5% of patients) include severe depression, neutropenia, and optic neuritis [56].

Currently, in many countries, access to the abovementioned interferons is very limited.

4. Surgical Treatment—Pars Plana Vitrectomy

Surgical treatment of uveitic ME remains a third-line therapy in most cases due to the significant risk of complications. However, pars plana vitrectomy should be considered for patients for whom the accumulation of inflammatory cytokines in the vitreous plays a dominant role. Some patients withstand vitrectomy surprisingly well, such as those with Fuch's syndrome and severe vitritis. Heterogeneous visual improvement after uveitis treatment applies to almost all therapeutic modalities but is especially significant for PPV patients. It can be difficult or even impossible to distinguish the effects of haze and edema reduction. In many cases, the change in visual acuity may be attributed to a reduction in inflammation. In fact, post-PPV CST may remain near baseline with possible intravitreal drug pharmacokinetic deterioration; for example, triamcinolone acetonide has an 18.6-day half-life in non-vitrectomized eyes versus only 3.2 days in vitrectomized eyes [57]. A direct comparison of general treatment and PPV favored systemic medication [58].

Ophthalmologists should be aware that in some patients with uveitis, inflammation can increase as a result of surgery, usually requiring increased doses of previously used drugs or the initiation of more extensive therapy. The risk–benefit ratio is often low, so the decision to perform PPV (e.g., in patients with inflammatory epiretinal membranes) should not be made too hastily.

The effect of PPV on the pharmacokinetics of intravitreal drugs is not well understood and has been investigated mainly in animal studies. However, it seems that the duration of therapeutic drug action in vitrectomized eyes is quite short, meaning that, in some cases, VEGF inhibitors may be administered as often as every two weeks [59]. Thus, PPV potentially increases the role of long-acting drugs such as dexamethasone implants in this patient group.

5. What to Consider When Choosing a Treatment

Many factors should be considered when choosing a treatment, since the effectiveness of treatments may vary from patient to patient. When deciding on a specific treatment method, the questions in Table 2 can be used in conjunction with the short pros/cons listed in Table 3.

Table 2. Questions facilitating the choice of treatment of uveitic ME.

Questions	Remarks
1. Has the patient been treated for ME? What were the effectiveness and complications of this treatment? Can the dose be adjusted to improve them? Is it better to repeat them, or does the response to this treatment suggest a need for change?	Previous treatment effects can be crucial when choosing an appropriate treatment regimen. Be sure to ask whether the patient has been treated previously by other ophthalmologists.
2. What complications should I especially avoid in this patient; for example, due to (a) advanced glaucoma changes, (b) age, (c) general diseases, (d) accompanying ocular changes, (e) the mental state of the patient, and/or (f) the expected compliance with medical recommendations?	ME is usually not the patient's only problem. Chronic use of steroids or interferons in general can be dangerous in terms of the patient's physical condition and mental health.
3. How often should I monitor and treat the patient—may I miss side effects or the need for additional treatment due to too infrequent follow-up visits?	IOP generally increases shortly after administration of periocular/intravitreal steroids; hence, after 1–2 weeks, it is worth checking the scale of this increase. VEGF inhibitors may not be effective for more than one month in many CME cases. This should be checked early in OCT, especially when starting therapy.
4. Is the patient a steroid responder for IOP?	If so, avoid local steroids unless pharmacological anti-glaucoma treatment is expected to be sufficient to normalize the IOP. In this case, do not start vitreous injections. Topical or posterior subtenon administration will be safer, although less effective, especially for the first option.
5. In the event of cataract formation, will it be safe to implant an artificial intraocular lens?	If not, try to avoid periocular/intravitreal steroids or intravitreal methotrexate. Administer oral steroids in carefully controlled doses.
6. Can a change in macular retinal morphology, especially a reduction in macular thickness, improve visual acuity?	Often, based on previously observed values, the patient's prognosis of improved vision can be estimated. Sometimes aggressive treatment will only improve the OCT cross-section.
7. Do both eyes need ME treatment, or is there a case for focusing on treating the eye with the best prognosis or only the one with edema?	Treatment of both eyes can often be easier with systemic medication.
8. Do the treatment results so far suggest that a combined therapy may be needed?	Systemic and local medications can complement each other, but they reduce the comfort of therapy.
9. Is inflammation still active? Is intense inflammation the main cause of the edema?	A cytokine storm is not a good time to focus on the ME itself. If the inflammation is not under control, ME treatment may be ineffective or have only short-term effects.

Table 3. Advantages and disadvantages of individual therapeutic options for uveitic ME. Signs in the table: -, +/-, +, ++, +++ are ranked from least to most favorable, respectively.

Treatment	Efficacy	Safety	Supported by EBM Data	Duration of Action (Single Administration)	Cost
Topical steroids	-	++	-	-	+++
Topical NSAIDs	-	+++	-	-	+++
Subconjunctival triamcinolone	+	++	+	+	+++
Periocular/subtenon triamcinolone/methyloprednisolone	++	+	++	+	+++
Intravitreal triamcinolone	+++	+	++	++	+++
Ozurdex®	+++	+	++	++	+
Iluvien®	+++	+	++	+++	+
Retisert®	+++	+	++	+++	+
Intravitreal VEGF inhibitors	+	++	+	+	++
Systemic steroids	++	+	++	-	+++
Systemic immunomodulatory drugs	++	++	+	+/-	+++
Systemic biologic treatments	++	++	+/-	+/-	++

5.1. Bilateral Versus Unilateral CME

Avoidance of general side effects from chronic medication use favors the choice of local treatment, especially when the edema affects only one eye. When ME is bilateral, the benefits of local treatment are less obvious, but it can still prevent many side effects. An ophthalmologist's decision not to treat both eyes simultaneously can also reduce the patient's comfort, leading to more frequent visits. Although there is no conclusive evidence of an unfavorable response to bilateral treatment with intravitreal injections in both eyes, ophthalmologists should be aware that the incidence of complications in uveitis is higher than with routine administration of VEGF inhibitors for age-related macular degeneration (AMD) [60]; hence, the simultaneous administration of intravitreal steroids in both eyes may not be the optimal choice.

5.2. Age

Treatment at a young age is a negative prognostic factor, although uveitic ME is more common at an advanced age [61]. Young people not only develop a more aggressive form of the disease more frequently, but due to their longer potential life spans, they may experience more frequent relapses, and their retinas, despite morphological changes, will have to function for longer periods. The treatment for young people may therefore have to be very intensive. ME, unlike retinal neovascularization, does not cause rapid and permanent vision-threatening changes; however, especially for young patients, quick initiation of effective treatment is highly recommended.

5.3. Phakic Status

This factor relates to the previous one. Although ME is more critical than the potential for cataract formation, it is important to remember that the lens removal procedure itself may exacerbate inflammation. Moreover, removing a young person's lens is a greater injury than it would be for a person with presbyopia. The use of multifocal intraocular lenses is not a good choice during cataract surgery in patients with uveitis, mainly for retinal reasons. Both for the patient and the ophthalmologist, because of the possible need to perform a vitrectomy, both epiretinal membrane (ERM) and internal limiting membrane (ILM) peeling are technically much more difficult in the presence of such lenses.

Ocular complications of cataract surgery in uveitis can be significant, and in some groups of patients—especially younger patients—even the use of biological drugs does not significantly reduce this risk [62]; thus, intravitreal steroids should be avoided if the prevention of cataract surgery is desirable.

5.4. Economy

The choice of treatment does not always depend on strictly medical reasons. The scope of reimbursement for particular methods, or their availability in a given country, may key factors determining the method of treatment.

5.5. Combined Treatment

In the absence of available evidence-based medicine (EBM) data on combination therapies for uveitic ME, there are no clear indications in this regard. Available drug interaction data should be consulted to avoid interactions that may cause side effects or show similar mechanisms of action. One possible option is the use of a local corticosteroid along with systemic immunomodulatory and/or biological therapy.

6. Conclusions

It is impossible to identify a single treatment regimen that covers most clinical situations in uveitic ME, and regimens can be error-prone in many cases; therefore, the author recommends asking some basic questions for each patient in order to choose a course of action that is both safe and effective. The questions should primarily relate to the patient's safety.

In many of the studies cited above, only half the patients responded well to ME treatment. Discussion with the patient is therefore important for deciding on an optimal treatment, including complex combined therapy, and this may take time and many attempts. If the patient is dissatisfied with the effects of a treatment and changes his doctor, previous attempts to identify an optimal treatment may be unnecessarily repeated. Cooperation based on trust is particularly important for treating ME, as it is for other chronic diseases. Acute treatment usually involves the use of steroids via various routes of administration, but long-term treatment should avoid steroid drugs because of their common side effects.

Funding: This research received no external funding.

Conflicts of Interest: The author declares no conflict of interest.

References

1. Acharya, N.R.; Thamm, V.M.; Esterberg, E.; Borkar, D.S.; Parker, J.V.; Vinoya, A.C.; Uchida, A. Incidence and prevalence of uveitis: Results from the Pacific Ocular Inflammation Study. *JAMA Ophthalmol.* **2013**, *131*, 1405–1412. [CrossRef]
2. Rao, N.A. Uveitis in developing countries. *Indian J. Ophthalmol.* **2013**, *61*, 253. [CrossRef]
3. Lardenoye, C.W.; van Kooij, B.; Rothova, A. Impact of macular edema on visual acuity in uveitis. *Ophthalmology* **2006**, *113*, 1446–1449. [CrossRef]
4. Massa, H.; Pipis, S.Y.; Adewoyin, T.; Vergados, A.; Patra, S.; Panos, G.D. Macular edema associated with non-infectious uveitis: Pathophysiology, etiology, prevalence, impact and management challenges. *Clin. Ophthalmol.* **2019**, *13*, 1761. [CrossRef]
5. Habot-Wilner, Z.; Trivizki, O.; Goldstein, M.; Kesler, A.; Shulman, S.; Horowitz, J.; Amer, R.; David, R.; Ben-Arie-Weintrob, Y.; Bakshi, E.; et al. Cat-scratch disease: Ocular manifestations and treatment outcome. *Acta Ophthalmol.* **2018**, *96*, e524–e532. [CrossRef] [PubMed]
6. Bernard, A.; Seve, P.; Abukhashabh, A.; Roure-Sobas, C.; Boibieux, A.; Denis, P.; Broussolle, C.; Mathis, T.; Kodjikian, L. Lyme-associated uveitis: Clinical spectrum and review of literature. *Eur. J. Ophthalmol.* **2020**, *30*, 874–885. [CrossRef]
7. Debiec, M.R.; Lindeke-Myers, A.T.; Shantha, J.G.; Bergstrom, C.S.; Hubbard, G.B.; Yeh, S. Outcomes of combination systemic and intravitreal antiviral therapy for acute retinal necrosis. *Ophthalmol. Retina* **2021**, *5*, 292–300. [CrossRef] [PubMed]
8. Agrawal, R.; Betzler, B.K.; Testi, I.; Mahajan, S.; Agarwal, A.; Gunasekeran, D.V.; Raje, D.; Aggarwal, K.; Murthy, S.I.; Westcott, M.; et al. The collaborative ocular tuberculosis study (COTS)-1: A multinational review of 447 patients with tubercular intermediate uveitis and panuveitis. *Ocul. Immunol. Inflamm.* **2020**, 1–11. [CrossRef] [PubMed]
9. Pichi, F.; Neri, P. Multimodal imaging patterns of posterior syphilitic uveitis: A review of the literature, laboratory evaluation and treatment. *Int. Ophthalmol.* **2020**, *40*, 1319–1329. [CrossRef] [PubMed]
10. Sahu, E.S.; Pal, B.; Sharma, T.; Biswas, J. Clinical profile, treatment, and visual outcome of ocular toxocara in a tertiary eye care centre. *Ocul. Immunol. Inflamm.* **2018**, *26*, 753–759. [CrossRef]

11. Yates, W.B.; Chiong, F.; Zagora, S.; Post, J.J.; Wakefield, D.; McCluskey, P. Ocular toxoplasmosis in a tertiary referral center in Sydney Australia: Clinical features, treatment, and prognosis. *Asia-Pac. J. Ophthalmol.* **2019**, *8*, 280–284. [CrossRef]
12. Petrushkin, H.; Rogers, D.; Pavesio, C. The use of topical non-steroidal anti-inflammatory drugs for uveitic cystoid macular edema. *Ocul. Immunol. Inflamm.* **2018**, *26*, 795–797. [CrossRef]
13. Radwan, A.E.; Arcinue, C.A.; Yang, P.; Artornsombudh, P.; Abu Al-Fadl, E.M.; Foster, C.S. Bromfenac alone or with single intravitreal injection of bevacizumab or triamcinolone acetonide for treatment of uveitic macular edema. *Graefes Arch. Clin. Exp. Ophthalmol.* **2013**, *251*, 1801–1806. [CrossRef] [PubMed]
14. Hariprasad, S.M.; Akduman, L.; Clever, J.A.; Ober, M.; Recchia, F.M.; Mieler, W.F. Treatment of cystoid macular edema with the new-generation NSAID nepafenac 0.1%. *Clin. Ophthalmol.* **2009**, *3*, 147–154. [CrossRef]
15. Kawali, A.; Srinivasan, S.; Mahendradas, P.; Shetty, R. Topical interferon in recurrent inflammatory macular edema following a cat bite. *Eur. J. Ophthalmol.* **2021**. [CrossRef]
16. Maleki, A.; Meese, H.; Sahawneh, H.; Foster, C.S. Progress in the understanding and utilization of biologic response modifiers in the treatment of uveitis. *Expert Rev. Clin. Immunol.* **2016**, *12*, 775–786. [CrossRef]
17. Maleki, A.; Stephenson, A.P.; Hajizadeh, F. Topical interferon alpha 2b in the treatment of refractory diabetic macular edema. *J. Ophthalmic Vis. Res.* **2020**, *15*, 453.
18. Couret, C.; Poinas, A.; Volteau, C.; Riche, V.P.; Le Lez, M.L.; Errera, M.H.; Creuzot-Garcher, C.; Baillif, S.; Kodjikian, L.; Ivan, C.; et al. Comparison of two techniques used in routine care for the treatment of inflammatory macular oedema, subconjunctival triamcinolone injection and intravitreal dexamethasone implant: Medical and economic importance of this randomized controlled trial. *Trials* **2020**, *21*, 1–13. [CrossRef]
19. Qu, Y.; Liu, X.-S.; Liang, A.-Y.; Xiao, J.-Y.; Zhao, C.; Gao, F.; Zhang, M.F. Subconjunctival injections of triamcinolone acetonide to treat uveitic macular edema. *Int. J. Ophthalmol.* **2020**, *13*, 1087–1091. [CrossRef]
20. Ying-Jiun, C.; Chee-Kuen, W.; Shatriah, I. Conjunctival necrosis following a subconjunctival injection of triamcinolone acetonide in a child. *Middle East Afr. J. Ophthalmol.* **2015**, *22*, 125–128.
21. Agrawal, S.; Agrawal, J.; Agrawal, T.P. Conjunctival ulceration following triamcinolone injection. *Am. J. Ophthalmol.* **2003**, *136*, 539–540. [CrossRef]
22. Smith, J.L.; McCrary, J.A.; Bird, A.C.; Kurstin, J.; Kulvin, S.M.; Skilling, F.D., Jr.; Acers, T.E.; Coston, T.O. Sub-tenon steroid injection for optic neuritis. *Trans. Am. Acad. Ophthalmol. Otolaryngol.* **1970**, *74*, 1249–1253.
23. McLean, E.B. Inadvertent injection of corticosteroid into the choroidal vasculature. *Am. J. Ophthalmol.* **1975**, *80*, 835–837. [CrossRef]
24. Inatani, M.; Iwao, K.; Kawaji, T.; Hirano, Y.; Ogura, Y.; Hirooka, K.; Shiraga, F.; Nakanishi, Y.; Yamamoto, H.; Negi, A.; et al. Intraocular pressure elevation after injection of triamcinolone acetonide: A multicenter retrospective case-control study. *Am. J. Ophthalmol.* **2008**, *145*, 676–681. [CrossRef]
25. Yang, Y.H.; Hsu, W.C.; Hsieh, Y.T. Anterior migration of triamcinolone acetonide after posterior subtenon injection for macular edema predisposes to intraocular pressure elevation. *Curr. Eye Res.* **2021**, *46*, 689–693. [CrossRef]
26. Maeda, Y.; Ishikawa, H.; Nishikawa, H.; Shimizu, M.; Kinoshita, T.; Ogihara, K.; Kitano, S.; Yamanaka, C.; Mitamura, Y.; Sugimoto, M.; et al. Intraocular pressure elevation after subtenon triamcinolone acetonide injection; Multicentre retrospective cohort study in Japan. *PLoS ONE* **2019**, *14*, e0226118. [CrossRef]
27. Kuo, H.K.; Lai, I.C.; Fang, P.C.; Teng, M.C. Ocular complications after a sub-tenon injection of triamcinolone acetonide for uveitis. *Chang Gung Med. J.* **2005**, *28*, 85–89.
28. Yeh, S.; Khurana, R.N.; Shah, M.; Henry, C.R.; Wang, R.C.; Kissner, J.M.; Ciulla, T.A.; Noronha, G.; PEACHTREE Study Investigators. Efficacy and safety of suprachoroidal CLS-TA for macular edema secondary to noninfectious uveitis: Phase 3 randomized trial. *Ophthalmology* **2020**, *127*, 948–955. [CrossRef]
29. Ozkiriş, A.; Erkiliç, K. Complications of intravitreal injection of triamcinolone acetonide. *Can. J. Ophthalmol.* **2005**, *40*, 63–68. [CrossRef]
30. Mishra, C.; Lalitha, P.; Rameshkumar, G.; Agrawal, R.; Balne, P.K.; Iswarya, M.; Kannan, N.B.; Ramasamy, K. Incidence of endophthalmitis after intravitreal injections: Risk factors, microbiology profile, and clinical outcomes. *Ocul. Immunol. Inflamm.* **2018**, *26*, 559–568. [CrossRef]
31. Dhoot, D.S.; Boucher, N.; Pitcher, J.D., 3rd; Saroj, N. Rates of suspected endophthalmitis following intravitreal injections in clinical practices in the United States. *Ophthalmic Surg. Lasers Imaging Retin.* **2021**, *52*, 312–318. [CrossRef]
32. Dodwell, D.G.; Krimmel, D.A.; de Fiebre, C.M. Sterile endophthalmitis rates and particle size analyses of different formulations of triamcinolone acetonide. *Clin. Ophthalmol.* **2015**, *9*, 1033–1040. [CrossRef]
33. Celik, N.; Khoramnia, R.; Auffarth, G.U.; Sel, S.; Mayer, C.S. Complications of dexamethasone implants: Risk factors, prevention, and clinical management. *Int. J. Ophthalmol.* **2020**, *13*, 1612–1620. [CrossRef]
34. Lowder, C.; Belfort, R., Jr.; Lightman, S.; Foster, C.S.; Robinson, M.R.; Schiffman, R.M.; Li, X.Y.; Cui, H.; Whitcup, S.M.; Ozurdex HURON Study Group. Dexamethasone intravitreal implant for noninfectious intermediate or posterior uveitis. *Arch. Ophthalmol.* **2011**, *129*, 545–553. [CrossRef]

35. Thorne, J.E.; Sugar, E.A.; Holbrook, J.T.; Burke, A.E.; Altaweel, M.M.; Vitale, A.T.; Acharya, N.R.; Kempen, J.H.; Jabs, D.A.; Multicenter Uveitis Steroid Treatment Trial Research Group. Periocular triamcinolone vs. intravitreal triamcinolone vs. intravitreal dexamethasone implant for the treatment of uveitic macular edema: The PeriOcular vs. INTravitreal corticosteroids for uveitic macular edema (POINT). Trial. *Ophthalmol.* **2019**, *126*, 283–295. [CrossRef]
36. Korobelnik, J.F.; Kodjikian, L.; Delcourt, C.; Gualino, V.; Leaback, R.; Pinchinat, S.; Velard, M.E. Two-year, prospective, multicenter study of the use of dexamethasone intravitreal implant for treatment of macular edema secondary to retinal vein occlusion in the clinical setting in France. *Graefes Arch. Clin. Exp. Ophthalmol.* **2016**, *254*, 2307–2318. [CrossRef]
37. Jaffe, G.J.; Pavesio, C.E.; Study Investigators. Effect of a fluocinolone acetonide insert on recurrence rates in noninfectious intermediate, posterior, or panuveitis: Three-year results. *Ophthalmology* **2020**, *127*, 1395–1404. [CrossRef]
38. Callanan, D.G.; Jaffe, G.J.; Martin, D.F.; Pearson, P.A.; Comstock, T.L. Treatment of posterior uveitis with a fluocinolone acetonide implant: Three-year clinical trial results. *Arch. Ophthalmol.* **2008**, *126*, 1191–1201.
39. Cho, H.; Madu, A. Etiology and treatment of the inflammatory causes of cystoid macular edema. *J. Inflamm. Res.* **2009**, *2*, 37. [CrossRef]
40. Monés, J.; Srivastava, S.K.; Jaffe, G.J.; Tadayoni, R.; Albini, T.A.; Kaiser, P.K.; Holz, F.G.; Korobelnik, J.F.; Kim, I.K.; Pruente, C.; et al. Risk of inflammation, retinal vasculitis, and retinal occlusion-related events with brolucizumab: Post hoc review of HAWK and HARRIER. *Ophthalmology* **2021**, *128*, 1050–1059. [CrossRef] [PubMed]
41. Staurenghi, G.; Lai, T.Y.Y.; Mitchell, P.; Wolf, S.; Wenzel, A.; Li, J.; Bhaumik, A.; Hykin, P.G.; PROMETHEUS Study Group. Efficacy and safety of ranibizumab 0.5 mg for the treatment of macular edema resulting from uncommon causes: Twelve-month findings from PROMETHEUS. *Ophthalmology* **2018**, *125*, 850–862. [CrossRef]
42. Kozak, I.; Shoughy, S.S.; Stone, D.U. Intravitreal antiangiogenic therapy of uveitic macular edema: A review. *J. Ocul. Pharmacol. Ther.* **2017**, *33*, 235–239. [CrossRef]
43. Rothova, A.; Berge, J.C.; Vingerling, J.R. Intravitreal aflibercept for treatment of macular oedema associated with immune recovery uveitis. *Acta Ophthalmol.* **2020**, *98*, e922. [CrossRef] [PubMed]
44. Taylor, S.R.; Habot-Wilner, Z.; Pacheco, P.; Lightman, S.L. Intraocular methotrexate in the treatment of uveitis and uveitic cystoid macular edema. *Ophthalmology* **2009**, *116*, 797–801. [CrossRef]
45. Taylor, S.R.; Banker, A.; Schlaen, A.; Couto, C.; Matthe, E.; Joshi, L.; Menezo, V.; Nguyen, E.; Tomkins-Netzer, O.; Bar, A.; et al. Intraocular methotrexate can induce extended remission in some patients in noninfectious uveitis. *Retina* **2013**, *33*, 2149–2154. [CrossRef]
46. Nguyen, Q.D.; Sadiq, M.A.; Soliman, M.K.; Agarwal, A.; Do, D.V.; Sepah, Y.J. The effect of different dosing schedules of intravitreal sirolimus, a mammalian target of rapamycin (mTOR) inhibitor, in the treatment of non-infectious uveitis (An American Ophthalmological Society Thesis). *Trans. Am. Ophthalmol. Soc.* **2016**, *114*, 3–4.
47. Babu, K.; Mahendradas, P. Medical Management of Uveitis—Current Trends. *Indian J. Ophthalmol.* **2013**, *61*, 277. [CrossRef]
48. Takeuchi, M.; Kanda, T.; Kaburaki, T.; Tanaka, R.; Namba, K.; Kamoi, K.; Maruyama, K.; Shibuya, E.; Mizuki, N. Real-world evidence of treatment for relapse of noninfectious uveitis in tertiary centers in Japan: A multicenter study. *Medicine* **2019**, *98*, e14668. [CrossRef]
49. Gómez-Gómez, A.; Loza, E.; Rosario, M.P.; Espinosa, G.; de Morales, J.M.G.R.; Herrera, J.M.; Muñoz-Fernández, S.; Rodríguez-Rodríguez, L.; Cordero-Coma, M.; Spanish Society of Ocular Inflammation (SEIOC). Efficacy and safety of immunomodulatory drugs in patients with non-infectious intermediate and posterior uveitis, panuveitis and macular edema: A systematic literature review. *Semin. Arthritis Rheum.* **2020**, *50*, 1299–1306. [CrossRef]
50. Kempen, J.H.; Daniel, E.; Gangaputra, S.; Dreger, K.; Jabs, D.A.; Kaçmaz, R.O.; Pujari, S.S.; Anzaar, F.; Foster, C.S.; Helzlsouer, K.J.; et al. Methods for identifying long-term adverse effects of treatment in patients with eye diseases: The systemic immunosuppressive therapy for eye diseases (SITE) cohort study. *Ophthalmic Epidemiol.* **2008**, *15*, 47–55. [CrossRef]
51. Levin, M.H.; Pistilli., M.; Daniel, E.; Gangaputra, S.S.; Nussenblatt, R.B.; Rosenbaum, J.T.; Suhler, E.B.; Thorne, J.E.; Foster, C.S.; Jabs, D.A.; et al. Systemic Immunosuppressive Therapy for Eye Diseases Cohort Study. Incidence of visual improvement in uveitis cases with visual impairment caused by macular edema. *Ophthalmology* **2014**, *121*, 588–595. [CrossRef]
52. Kempen, J.H.; Daniel, E.; Dunn, J.P.; Foster, C.S.; Gangaputra, S.; Hanish, A.; Helzlsouer, K.J.; Jabs, D.A.; Kaçmaz, R.O.; Levy-Clarke, G.A.; et al. Overall and cancer related mortality among patients with ocular inflammation treated with immunosuppressive drugs: Retrospective cohort study. *BMJ* **2009**, *339*, 89–92. [CrossRef] [PubMed]
53. Barry, R.J.; Tallouzi, M.O.; Bucknall, N.; Mathers, J.M.; Murray, P.I.; Calvert, M.J.; Moore, D.J.; Denniston, A.K. Anti-tumour necrosis factor biological therapies for the treatment of uveitic macular oedema (UMO) for non-infectious uveitis. *Cochrane Database Syst. Rev.* **2018**, *12*, CD012577. [CrossRef]
54. Steeples, L.R.; Spry, P.; Lee, R.W.J.; Carreño, E. Adalimumab in refractory cystoid macular edema associated with birdshot chorioretinopathy. *Int. Ophthalmol.* **2018**, *38*, 1357–1362. [CrossRef]
55. Mackensen, F.; Jakob, E.; Springer, C.; Dobner, B.C.; Wiehler, U.; Weimer, P.; Rohrschneider, K.; Fiehn, C.; Max, R.; Storch-Hagenlocher, B.; et al. Interferon versus methotrexate in intermediate uveitis with macular edema: Results of a randomized controlled clinical trial. *Am. J. Ophthalmol.* **2013**, *156*, 478–486. [CrossRef]
56. Bodaghi, B.; Gendron, G.; Wechsler, B.; Terrada, C.; Cassoux, N.; Huong, D.L.T.; Lemaitre, C.; Fradeau, C.; LeHoang, P.; Piette, J.C. Efficacy of interferon alpha in the treatment of refractory and sight threatening uveitis: A retrospective monocentric study of 45 patients. *Br. J. Ophthalmol.* **2007**, *91*, 335–339. [CrossRef]

57. Beer, P.M.; Bakri, S.J.; Singh, R.J.; Liu, W.; Peters, G.B., 3rd; Miller, M. Intraocular concentration and pharmacokinetics of triamcinolone acetonide after a single intravitreal injection. *Ophthalmology* **2003**, *110*, 681–686. [CrossRef]
58. Shalaby, O.; Saeed, A.; Elmohamady, M.N. Immune modulator therapy compared with vitrectomy for management of complicated intermediate uveitis: A prospective, randomized clinical study. *Arq. Bras. Oftalmol.* **2020**, *83*, 402–409. [CrossRef]
59. Edington, M.; Connolly, J.; Chong, N.V. Pharmacokinetics of intravitreal anti-VEGF drugs in vitrectomized versus non-vitrectomized eyes. *Expert Opin. Drug Metab. Toxicol.* **2017**, *13*, 1217–1224. [CrossRef]
60. VanderBeek, B.L.; Bonaffini, S.G.; Ma, L. The association between intravitreal steroids and post-injection endophthalmitis rates. *Ophthalmology* **2015**, *122*, 2311–2315.e1. [CrossRef]
61. Prieto-Del-Cura, M.; González-Guijarro, J.J. Risk factors for ocular complications in adult patients with uveitis. *Eur. J. Ophthalmol.* **2020**, *30*, 1381–1389. [CrossRef]
62. Bolletta, E.; Coassin, M.; Iannetta, D.; Mastrofilippo, V.; Aldigeri, R.; Invernizzi, A.; de Simone, L.; Gozzi, F.; De Fanti, A.; Cappella, M.; et al. Cataract surgery with intraocular lens implantation in juvenile idiopathic arthritis-associated uveitis: Outcomes in the era of biological therapy. *J. Clin. Med.* **2021**, *10*, 2437. [CrossRef] [PubMed]

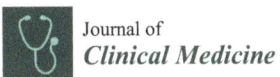

Review

Current Management Options in Irvine–Gass Syndrome: A Systemized Review

Michał Orski [1,*] and Maciej Gawęcki [2]

1 Department of Ophthalmology, Ludwik Rydygier Memorial Hospital, Złotej Jesieni 1, 31-826 Krakow, Poland
2 Dobry Wzrok Ophthalmological Clinic, Kliniczna 1B/2, 80-402 Gdansk, Poland; maciej@gawecki.com
* Correspondence: orski.michal@gmail.com

Abstract: Irvine–Gass syndrome (IGS) remains one of the most common complications following uneventful cataract surgery. In most cases, macular edema (ME) in IGS is benign, self-limiting, and resolves spontaneously without visual impairment; however, persistent edema and refractory cases may occur and potentially deteriorate visual function. Despite the relatively high prevalence of IGS, no solid management guidelines exist. We searched the PUBMED database for randomized clinical trials (RCT) or case series of at least 10 cases published since 2000 evaluating different treatment strategies in patients with cystoid macular edema (CME). The search revealed 28 papers that fulfilled the inclusion criteria with only seven RCTs. The scarceness of material makes it impossible to formulate strong recommendations for the treatment of IGS. Clinical practice and theoretical background support topical non-steroidal anti-inflammatory drugs (NSAIDs) as the first-line therapy. Invasive procedures, such as periocular steroids, intravitreal corticosteroids, and anti-vascular endothelial growth factor (anti-VEGF), are usually applied in prolonged or refractory cases. Results of novel applications of subthreshold micropulse laser (SML) are also promising and should be studied carefully in terms of the safety profile and cost effectiveness. Early initiation of invasive treatment for providing better functional results must be examined in further research.

Keywords: Irvine–Gass syndrome; cystoid macular edema; pseudophakic macular edema; NSAIDs corticosteroids; anti-VEGF; subthreshold diode micropulse

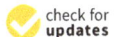

Citation: Orski, M.; Gawęcki, M. Current Management Options in Irvine–Gass Syndrome: A Systemized Review. *J. Clin. Med.* **2021**, *10*, 4375. https://doi.org/10.3390/jcm10194375

Academic Editors: María Isabel López-Gálvez and Giacinto Triolo

Received: 9 August 2021
Accepted: 18 September 2021
Published: 25 September 2021

Publisher's Note: MDPI stays neutral with regard to jurisdictional claims in published maps and institutional affiliations.

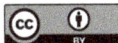

Copyright: © 2021 by the authors. Licensee MDPI, Basel, Switzerland. This article is an open access article distributed under the terms and conditions of the Creative Commons Attribution (CC BY) license (https://creativecommons.org/licenses/by/4.0/).

1. Introduction

Postoperative cystoid macular edema (CME) remains one of the most common complications of intraocular surgery. It is defined as a presence of intraretinal fluid (IF) spaces or central macular thickening (CMF) in optical coherence tomography (OCT) examination [1]. Irvine–Gass syndrome (IGS), sometimes named pseudophakic cystoid macular edema (PCME), is a cystoid macular edema that develops following uneventful cataract surgery. It was first described in 1953 by Irvine and studied using fluorescein angiography (FA) by Gass and Norton in 1966 [2,3]. Irvine–Gass syndrome remains the most common cause of decreased visual acuity after uneventful cataract surgery [4]. In most cases, no treatment is indicated as it resolves spontaneously, but persistent edema may also occur. Hunter et al. reported that 26.8% of eyes with pseudophakic CME did not recover 6/6 vision [5].

The incidence of Irvine–Gass syndrome varies among studies and is highly dependent on the diagnostic criteria [6]. Diagnosis is made based on clinical findings along with visual impairment or based on the presence of FA leakage or IF on OCT scans. OCT shows cystic intraretinal spaces on high-resolution cross-sectional scans of the macula that can be accompanied by mild photoreceptors detachment [4,7]. The early phases of FA show macular leakage, and as FA helps to rule out other causes of macular edema (ME), it remains a gold standard as a diagnostic tool [8] when used with the OCT.

Clinically significant CME impairing patients' vision is found in 1–2% of patients with its peak 6 weeks following surgery, but subclinical CME can be seen in about 30%

of patients in FA and up to 40% in OCT [4,7,9]. The risk factors include the presence of epiretinal membrane, history of uveitis, diabetes mellitus, and use of topical medications for glaucoma.

Several models have been considered, but multifactorial inflammatory origin seems to play a major role in the pathophysiology of Irvine–Gass syndrome. Surgical manipulation causes significant release of inflammatory mediators, including arachidonic acid, cytokines, lysozyme, and vascular endothelial growth factor (VEGF). The inflammatory cascade impairs the blood–aqueous and blood–retinal barriers and promotes vascular permeability [10,11]. Fluid accumulates in the outer plexiform and inner nuclear layers, creating cystic intraretinal spaces that coalesce to larger fluid cavities [6]. Prolonged CME may cause lamellar holes and persistent subretinal fluid.

To date, there are no uniform recommendations for the treatment of Irvine–Gass syndrome, and variable strategies are employed. This review aims to present the most important contemporary therapeutic strategies in IGS based on available modern literature.

2. Material and Methods

The PUBMED database was searched for a combination of phrases including the terms Irvin–Gass syndrome or pseudophakic cystoid edema and steroids, intravitreal steroids, periocular steroids, triamcinolone, sub-tenon triamcinolone, dexamethasone, OZURDEX®, fluocinolone, non-steroidal anti-inflammatory drugs, anti-VEGF, aflibercept, ranibizumab, bevacizumab, carbonic anhydrase inhibitors, and acetazolamide.

Only randomized clinical trials or case series of at least 10 cases published since 2000 were included in the analysis and presented in the following tables. Reports using smaller samples were quoted only if larger studies were scarce or unavailable for the specific treatment modality.

The search revealed 28 articles, including 7 RCTs on the subject, that fulfilled inclusion criteria. Results were grouped according to the analyzed treatment modality.

If a treatment modality was not analyzed in a larger case series or RCT, results were presented descriptively.

3. Results

3.1. Non-Steroidal Anti-Inflammatory Drugs (NSAID)

The search revealed seven studies, including two RCTs, that met inclusion criteria analyzing the efficacy of NSAID eye drops in the treatment of IGS. The results of those studies are presented in Table 1. All the studies show functional and morphological improvement, although most patients still present some visual deficit at the end of the treatment. The latest studies favor topical nepafenac compared to other NSAID eye drops. No significant adverse events associated with the use of NSAIDs were reported in any of the studies.

Table 1. Results of the studies analyzing the efficacy of NSAID in the treatment of IGS that involved at least 10 cases and were published since 2000.

No	Study	No of Eyes	Duration of CME	Study Design	Results
1	Giarmoukakis et al., 2020 [12]	21 eyes treated with TN 0.3%	Acute (<4 months) and chronic (>4 months)	Prospective, clinic-based, non-randomized case-series	BCVA improvement from 0.49 ± 0.36 logMAR to 0.36 ± 0.42 logMAR at the last follow-up visit ($p < 0.005$). CRT decreased from 450.40 ± 90.74 μm at baseline to 354.60 ± 81.49 μm ($p < 0.05$)
2	Guclu et al., 2019 [13]	62 The IVD group included 32 eyes, and the TN group included 30 eyes	2 months	Retrospective; two arms: IVD: 32 patients, TN 0.1%: 30 patients; changes in BCVA, CMT at baseline, 1 month, 3 months, 6 months	Results at 6 months: BCVA change in ETDRS letters for IVD from 25 ± 11.8 to 49.3 ± 6.8 versus 20.9 ± 9.3 to 32.9 ± 7.3 for TN; CMT reduction from 522.7 ± 120.7 μm to 266.1 ± 53.4 μm for IVD versus 501.2 ± 104.2 to 364.9 ± 56.3 μm) for TN; statistically significantly better improvements for IVD than TN
3	Sengupta et al., 2018 [14]	69	Acute, precise duratio not defined	Retrospective; combined topical prednisolone QID for 6 weeks and TN for at least 6 weeks QID; evaluation of effect at 6 weeks; success criterion: BCVA 6/9 and CMT ≤300 mm; definition of any success: anything less than success and reduction of CMT by 150 mm	Success achieved in 37 eyes (54%) and any success in 55 eyes (80%) at 6 weeks
4	Yuksel et al., 2017 [15]	24 TA arm 24 TN arm	Mean duration 4.8 ± 5.0 weeks for TA and 4.5 ± 3.1 weeks for TN	Prospective; two arms: TA and TN; changes in CMT and BCVA at 6 months	Significant reduction of CMT and improvement of BCVA in both groups; BCVA change from 0.99 ± 0.62 logMAR to 0.63 ± 0.74 for TA and from 0.84 ± 0.65 to 0.37 ± 0.48 for TN reduction of CMT from 513.3 to 318.9 mm in TA arm and from 483.7 to 278.0 mm in TN arm; BCVA statistically better improvement in the TN arm
5	Warren et al., 2010 [16]	39	Chronic 6 months, mean 9.4 months	RCT; evaluation of the effect of adding topical NSAID in IGS; Design: IVT and IVB at study entry; IVB repeated after 1 month; afterward randomization to topical diclofenac 0.1% or ketorolac 0.4% or nepafenac 0.1% or bromfenac 0.09% or placebo for 16 weeks; evaluation at 16 weeks	Significant reduction of CMT compared with placebo for TN and topical bromfenac; improvement of BCVA for nepafenac only (by 19%)

Table 1. Cont.

No	Study	No of Eyes	Duration of CME	Study Design	Results
6	Hariprasad et al., 2009 [17]	22 eyes with pseudophakic and uveitic CME, including 13 with chronic IGS and 3 with acute IGS (20 patients) treated with TN 0.1%)	Acute IGS < 6 months Chronic IGS > 6 months	Retrospective multicenter review of 22 CME cases treated with TN 0.1% (six with concomitant prednisolone acetate 1%); duration of the follow up from 6 weeks to 6 months	BCVA improvement in 2 acute IGS (from 0.4 logMAR to 0.18 logMAR and from 0.3 logMAR to 0.14 logMAR). CRT reduction from 448 to 211 mm and from 306 to 284 mm. Morphological improvement in the third acute case: reduction of CMT from 380 to 236 mm, but no BCVA change due to retinal degeneration; mean BCVA improvement in the chronic group from 0.63 ± 0.33 logMAR to 0.30 ± 0.16 logMAR and mean CMT reduction from 451 ± 145.7 to 273 ± 80.8 mm
7	Rho 2003 [18]	34: Diclofenac 18 Ketorolac 16	Acute: 4.2 ± 1.4 months for ketorolac group and 4.0 ± 1.4 months for diclofenac group	Randomized prospective; evaluation of effects of topical diclofenac sodium 0.1% versus ketorolac tromethamine 0.5% in the treatment of IGS; evaluation at 26 weeks	BCVA change ketorolac: from $20/160 \pm 75.8$ to $20/58 \pm 94.1$ diclofenac: from $20/173 \pm 94$ to $20/49 \pm 56.8$ Reduction of CME at 26 weeks: diclofenac 16 (89%), ketorolac 14 (88%); elimination of CME at 26 weeks: diclofenac 14 (78%), ketorolac 12 (75%); no significant difference between the drugs

RCT: randomized controlled trial; IGS: Irvine–Gass syndrome; ME: macular edema; IVD: intravitreal dexamethasone implant; FA: fluorescein angiography; IVB: intravitreal bevacizumab; CMT: central macular thickness; TA: triamcinolone acetonide; TN: topical nepafenac; BCVA: best-corrected visual acuity; CME: cystoid macular edema; QID–quater in die.

3.2. Carbonic Anhydrase Inhibitors (CAI)

The search revealed only 2 studies that analyzed the additional effect of 250–500 mg of oral acetazolamide compared to that from topical NSAIDs or corticosteroids alone (Table 2). Both papers present better functional and morphological results of combined NSAID with or without corticosteroid plus CAI. Both papers present better functional and morphological results of NSAID combined with CAI. No data evaluating the potential role of topical CAIs were found.

Table 2. Results of the studies analyzing the efficacy of CAI in the treatment of IGS that involved at least 10 cases and were published since 2000.

No	Study	No of Eyes	Duration of CME	Study Design	Results
1	Curkovic et al., 2005 [19]	14 7–0.1% topical dexamethason + topical flurbiprofen (group 1) 7–0.1% topical dexamethason + topical flurbiprofen plus acetazolamide 250 mg 3× (group 2)	Not defined	RCT, the efficacy of oral acetazolamide of 250 mg TID in addition to topical dexamethasone and flurbiprofen	Complete resolution of CME in 86% of eyes receiving acetazolamide (plus the topical NSAID-steroid combination) vs. 29% in the control group who received topical dexamethasone and flurbiprofen alone BCVA change significantly better in group 2 from 0.32 ± 0.1 to 0.67 ± 0.1 versus 0.34 ± 0.12 to 0.53 ± 0.14 in group 1 (Snellen fraction)
2	Catier et al., 2005 [20]	16	5 months	Retrospective review 250–500 mg of acetazolamide per day associated with topical NSAID or steroids	Mean improvement of BCVA from 20/100 (0.7 ± 0.28 Log MAR) to 20/40 (+0.3 ± 0.2 Log MAR) and reduction of CMT from 599.67 ± 174.17 mm to 264.69 ± 106.59 mm; complete resolution in 87.5% cases and in 100% of cases treated by a combination of acetazolamide, NSAIDs and steroids

CT: randomized controlled trial; IGS: Irvine–Gass syndrome; CMT: central macular thickness; NSAID: non-steroidal anti-inflammatory drugs; BCVA: best-corrected visual acuity; CME: cystoid macular edema; mo—month; TID—ter in die.

3.3. Corticosteroids

3.3.1. Topical Corticosteroids

The search revealed only two studies that analyzed the additional effect of topical corticosteroids compared to NSAIDs alone. The results are presented in Table 3 and do not provide an unequivocal answer whether any additional effect exists: possible benefits are advocated in the Heier et al. study [21] but not confirmed in the study by Singal et al. [22].

Table 3. Results of the studies analyzing the efficacy of the addition of topical corticosteroids to NSAID in the treatment of IGS that involved at least 10 cases and were published since 2000.

No	Study	No of Eyes	Duration of CME	Study Design	Results
1	Heier et al., 2000 [21]	28 (26 completed the study)	Acute: 21–90 days after surgery	RCT, patients randomized to topical therapy with ketorolac (group K), prednisolone (group P), or ketorolac and prednisolone combination therapy (group C) QID. Follow up, 3 months.	BCVA improvements (Snellen lines): 1.6 in group K, 1.21 in group P, and 3.8 in group C. Treatment of acute, visually significant pseudophakic CME with ketorolac and prednisolone combination therapy appears to offer benefits over monotherapy with either agent alone
2	Singal et al., 2004 [22]	10 Ketorolac: 4 Ketorolac and tromethamine: 6	6 weeks and longer	RCT: prospective double-masked randomized controlled trial. 10 patients were randomly assigned to receive either 0.5% ketorolac tromethamine plus placebo or 0.5% ketorolac tromethamine plus 1% prednisolone acetate; follow up, 90 days	No statistically significant difference was found in the outcome between patients who received ketorolac and those who received ketorolac plus prednisolone for acute or chronic CME

RCT: randomized controlled trial; IGS: Irvine–Gass syndrome; CMT: central macular thickness NSAID: non-steroidal anti-inflammatory drugs; BCVA: best-corrected visual acuity; CME: cystoid macular edema.

3.3.2. Periocular Corticosteroids

The search revealed only three papers fulfilling the search criteria. The results of these studies are presented in Table 4. All are retrospective analyses and present significant improvement of both macular morphology and BCVA after sub-tenon injection of triamcinolone acetonide (STT) in IGS patients. A study by Kuley et al. [23] compared the effects of STT and IVT in a large sample but did not show a significant difference in final effect depending on the drug administration route.

Table 4. Results of the studies analyzing the efficacy of periocular corticosteroids in the treatment of IGS that involved at least 10 cases and were published since 2000.

No	Study	No of Eyes	Duration of CME	Study Design	Results
1	Kuley et al., 2021 [23]	50 STT 45 IVT	Not stated	Retrospective; comparison of resolution of IGS in two arms: 2 mg IVT or 40 mg STT at 1, 3, and 6 months	Insignificant difference in BCVA improvement: 2.3 lines in the IVT group and 2.4 lines in the STT group; CMT reduction was significantly better in the IVT group at month 1 (255 mm vs. 187 mm), but the difference was not present at month 3 (214 mm vs. 212 mm) and month 6 (176 mm vs. 207 mm); ocular hypertension managed by topical therapy in 7% of eyes in the IVT group and 12% of eyes in the STT group
2	Erden et al., 2019 [24]	21	Not stated	Retrospective; patients treatment naïve; injection of 40 mg of STT; minimum follow up 6 months	Significant improvement of mean BCVA from 0.71 ± 0.23 logMAR to 0.19 ± 0.06 logMAR and significant reduction of CMT from 431 ± 136 mm to 299 ± 66 mm at 6 months
3	Tsai et al., 2018 [25]	17	57.9 ± 50.1 days (range: 21–178 days).	Retrospective; 40 mg of STT; evaluation of BCVA and CMT at 1 and 3 months	Change of logMAR BCVA from baseline 0.75 ± 0.23 to 0.50 ± 0.20 at month 1 and 0.40 ± 0.20 at month 3. Change of CMT from baseline 446 ± 107 mm to 354 ± 90 mm at month 1 and 300 ± 58 mm at month 3. Insignificant rise of IOP < 21 mm Hg

RCT: randomized controlled trial; IGS: Irvine–Gass syndrome; ME: macular edema; IVD: intravitreal dexamethasone implant; FA: fluorescein angiography; IVB: intravitreal bevacizumab; IVT—intravitreal triamcinolone; CMT: central macular thickness; TA: triamcinolone acetonide; STT: sub-tenon triamcinolone; IOP: intraocular pressure; BCVA: best-corrected visual acuity.

3.3.3. Intravitreal Corticosteroid

In the search, we found eight larger reports published since 2000[t] that are presented in Table 5. The search revealed only two larger studies evaluating the efficacy of IVT in IGS (listed in Table 5). However, randomized controlled trials of IVT are missing. In addition, transient effects and the need for repeated injections remain a challenge [26]. Most high-quality studies on the use of intravitreal corticosteroids in IGS are focused on the use of an intravitreal dexamethasone implant (IVD) of 700 micrograms, commercially used under the name OZURDEX® (five studies). One study associated the results of IGS treatment with either IVD, IVT, or anti-VEGF to the time point of initiation of treatment [27]. Most of the patients were treated with IVD. All the listed studies demonstrated significant letter gains after intravitreal corticosteroid therapy without serious adverse events. Few cases of intraocular pressure rise were controlled with topical anti-glaucoma medication. The study by Sharma and his group showed that early initiation of intravitreal treatment in IGS provides better functional results [27]. The use of the a fluocinolone implant was not tested on a larger sample; however, available reports confirm its efficacy in the resolution of IGS in recurrent cases [28].

Table 5. Results of the studies analyzing the efficacy of intravitreal corticosteroids in the treatment of IGS that involved at least 10 cases and were published since 2000.

No	Study	No of Eyes	Duration of CME (Months)	Study Design	Results
1	Sharma et al., 2020 [27]	79	Less than 14 weeks	Retrospective; evaluation of the effect of IVD or IVT or anti-VEGF in IGS; evaluation at 12 months	IVD in 73.4% of eyes as initial therapy; switch from anti-VEGF to dexamethasone in 54.5% of cases; BCVA gain and CMT reduction 16.7 ± 12.9 letters and 336.7 ± 191.7 mm in patients treated within 4 weeks from diagnosis versus 5.2 ± 9.2 letters and 160.1 ± 153.1 mm for patients treated after 14 weeks from diagnosis; IOP rise in 3 patients after IVD controlled with topical medications
2	Altintas et al., 2019 [29]	10	Minimum 3 months	Retrospective; IGS resistant to topical treatment and IVB; implantation of IVD	Significant improvement of mean BCVA from 0.69 ± 0.19 logMAR to 0.19 ± 0.05 logMAR and significant reduction of mean CMT from 476.13 ± 135.13 mm to 268.38 ± 31.35 mm; mean number of IVD: 1.44 ± 0.89

Table 5. Cont.

No	Study	No of Eyes	Duration of CME (Months)	Study Design	Results
3	Bellocq et al., 2017 [30]	100	Mean 4.8 months	Retrospective multicenter national case series of 100 eyes receiving IVD for post-surgical macular edema	Mean improvement in BCVA was 9.6 ± 10.6 letters at month 6 and 10.3 ± 10.7 letters at month 12; BCVA gains of 15 or more letters noted in 32.5% cases and 37.5% cases at months 6 and 12, respectively; mean reduction in CSMT of 135.2 mm and 160.9 mm at months 6 and 12, respectively 37% of patients required only one IVD during the first year and experienced no recurrence of the macular edema in a follow-up period of greater than 1 year
4	Mayer et al., 2015 [31]	23	Mean 5.4 months (range 2–8)	Prospective; treatment with IVD; evaluation of BCVA and CMT at 12 months	Significant improvement of mean BCVA from 30.2 ± 4.3 letters to 50.4 ± 4.9 letters and decrease of CMT from 520.8 ± 71.4 mm to 232.7 ± 26.6 mm; no relevant adverse effects were noted
5	Zamil 2015 [32]	11	Mean 7.7 months (range 6–10)	Retrospective; single IVD; evaluation at 6 months	Significant mean BCVA improvement from 0.58 ± 0.17 logMAR to 0.21 ± 0.15 logMAR and reduction of mean CMT from 513.8 mm to 308.0 mm; no adverse events were noted
6	Sevim et al., 2012 [33]	IVT: 20; PPV: 19	6 months and longer	Retrospective; comparison of BCVA and CMT in two arms: IVT and PPV; evaluation at 12 months	BCVA change at 12 months: IVT: from 0.75 ± 0.23 logMAR to 0.45 ± 0.23 logMAR PPV: 0.78 ± 0.25 logMAR to 0.51 ± 0.21 logMAR; CMT change at 12 months: IVT: 536.00 ± 52.04 mm to 313.15 ± 44.30 mm PPV: 524.05 ± 63.49 mm to 326.31 ± 72.88 mm; significant improvement of BCVA and reduction of CMT at 12 months; no significant difference between the arms at 12 months; temporary
7	Williams et al., 2009 [34]	41	90 days and longer	RCT; CME secondary to uveitis or IGS, persistent 90 days; Three arms IVD (700 mg) or intravitreal dexamethasone 350 mg or observation	Improvement of at least 10 ETDRS letters at day 90: 41.7% in 350 mg group 53.8% in 700 mg group 7.1% in observed group; significant reduction of leakage on FA in treated patients; intraocular pressure rise of 10 mm Hg or more in 5 of 13 patients in the 700 mg group and in 1 of 12 patients in the 350 mg group, controlled by topical medication
8	Koutsandrea et al., 2007 [35]	14	Longer than 6 months	Retrospective; 14 eyes treated with IVT; follow up 12 months	Improvement of BCVA from mean 2.22 ± 0.16 to 0.36 ± 0.24 (decimal values) at 12 months; improvement of BCVA in 11 cases, stable in 2 cases and worsening in 1 case; reduction of CMT from mean 434.93 to 402.79 ± 162.22 mm; reduction of CMT in 11 cases and increase in 3 cases; increase in mf-ERG values; minor increase in IOP; topical IOP-lowering drops in 3 patients

RCT: randomized controlled trial; IGS: Irvine–Gass syndrome; CME: cystoid macular edema; IVD: intravitreal dexamethasone implant (700 mg); IVT: intravitreal triamcinolone; PPV: pars plana vitrectomy; FA: fluorescein angiography; IVB: intravitreal bevacizumab; CMT: central macular thickness; mf-ERG: multifocal electroretinogram; BCVA: best-corrected visual acuity.

3.4. Anti-VEGF

The search revealed six larger studies analyzing the effects of different anti-VEGF medications in the treatment of IGS: four studies employed intravitreal bevacizumab (IVB), one dedicated to intravitreal ranibizumab (IVR) and one compared the efficacy of the available three agents: aflibercept, ranibizumab, and bevacizumab. Results of those studies are presented in Table 6 and show significant visual and morphological improvements for all the available anti-VEGF medications without serious adverse effects. Intravitreal aflibercept (IVA), a more recent anti-VEGF agent, has been tried in the treatment of IGS, but except for one comparative study listed in Table 6, only case reports have been published on the use of aflibercept [36].

Anecdotal reports of combined intravitreal anti-VEGF and corticosteroids in the treatment of IGS exist, but these are only case reports, not larger trials [37]. Therefore, it is difficult to judge the additional effect of those drugs compared to anti-VEGF therapy alone in IGS.

Table 6. Results of the studies analyzing the efficacy of intravitreal anti-VEGF agents in the treatment of IGS that involved at least 10 cases and were published since 2000.

No	Study	No of Eyes	Duration of CME	Study Design	Results
1	Akay et al., 2020 [38]	59; IVB: 22, IVR: 19, IVA: 18	Not stated; refractory to topical treatment	Retrospective, controlled consecutive case series; comparison of functional and morphological results of treatment among 3 agents at 6 months	BCVA change: IVB: 0.96 ± 0.18 to 0.23 ± 0.19 IVR: 0.89 ± 0.23 to 0.19 ± 0.18 IVA: 0.94 ± 0.22 to 0.21 ± 0.08 CMT change: IVB: 555.5 ± 238.5 mm to 213.5 ± 21.1 mm IVR: 553.5 ± 125.5 mm to 226.6 ± 18.1 mm IVA: 540.0 ± 64.5 mm to 227.7 ± 39.5 mm No of injections: IVB: 1.8 ± 0.7 IVR: 2.0 ± 0.6 IVA: 1.8 ± 0.7 No significant difference in results of treatment and number of injections needed among the three agents
2	Staurenghi et al., 2018 [39]	40	3 months and longer	RCT; IVR 0.5 mg for IGS/aphakic eyes; one injection of IVR at baseline, then PRN regimen	Letter gain at month 2: 8.5 in the IVR group and 4.1 in the sham group (significant difference) At month 12: letter gain 14.5 vs. 10.5; minor adverse events related to injection (e.g., conjunctival hemorrhage)
3	Arevalo et al., 2009 [40]	36	3 months and longer	Retrospective; at least 1 injection of IVB in a dose of 1.25 or 2.5 mg; follow up 12 months	Improvement of BCVA of 2 ETDRS lines in 72.2%; none of the eyes worsened; mean BCVA change from 0.96 to 0.62 logMAR; CMT change from 499.9 to 286.1 mm; Mean no. of injections: 2.7
4	Barone et al., 2009 [41]	10	Mean 17.5 weeks (range 11–24)	At least one IVB 1.25 mg; evaluation of BCVA and CMT at 6 months	BCVA improvement in all eyes; Mean BCVA change from 20/80 to 20/32; mean CMT change from 546.8 to 228.7 mm
5	Spitzer 2008 [42]	16	Mean 14 weeks (range 3–84 weeks)	Retrospective case series; 1.25 mg of IVB; evaluation of BCVA change and CMT change	BCVA improvement by 2 ETDRS letters in 1 eye, unchanged in 12 eyes and worsened in 2 eyes; reduction in CMT by more than 10% in 9 eyes
6	Arevalo et al., 2007 [43]	25	Not stated	Retrospective; IVB of 1.25 or 2.5 mg; mean follow up 32 weeks	Improvement of BCVA of 2 ETDRS lines in 71.4%; none of the eyes worsened; mean BCVA change from 0.92 to 0.50 logMAR; CMT change from 466.3 to 264.5 mm; 28.6% of eyes required a second injection, and 14.3% required a third injection

RCT: randomized controlled trial; IGS: Irvine–Gass syndrome; CME: cystoid macular edema; IVB: intravitreal bevacizumab; IVR: intravitreal ranibizumab; IVA: intravitreal aflibercept; IVD: intravitreal dexamethasone implant (700 mg); BCVA: best-corrected visual acuity; CMT: central macular thickness.

3.5. Subthreshold Micropulse Laser (SML)

A photostimulation process with repetitive short pulses delivered at a subthreshold mode allows foveal treatment with no damage compared to conventional laser treatments. The benefits of SML in the treatment of different macular disorders such as central serous chorioretinopathy (CSC), diabetic macular edema (DME), and macular edema secondary to retinal vein occlusion (RVO) were shown in many studies [44,45].

In 2020, Verdina et al. published the first results of the treatment of refractory postoperative CME with subthreshold micropulse yellow laser in 10 eyes of 10 patients [46]. Five eyes of five patients had Irvine–Gass syndrome. A retrospective analysis showed improvement of BCVA and CMT in all patients, and the effects were maintained through 1, 2, 3, and 6 months. The treatment used a 577 nm subliminal laser photo-stimulation treatment with 7×7 grids with confluent spots and a 5% duty cycle. Treatment was targeted at whole edematous retina, including the foveal center. The study demonstrated complete resolution of retinal edema and improvement of BCVA in all patients with no side effects. The mean number of laser treatments was 1.3.

3.6. Laser Photocoagulation (LPC)

No studies of LPC in IGS published after 2000 were found in the PUBMED database. Previous studies reported a beneficial effect of modified GRID protocol for IGS; however, these were not controlled studies [47].

3.7. Other Treatments

Interferon alfa was administered for IGS in a small case series of four eyes refractory to topical treatment [48]. A 3 million IU/day dose was injected subcutaneously for 4 weeks and tapered thereafter. Improvement was achieved in three cases without any side effects. Topical treatment of chronic refractory IGS with interferon alfa was also reported in a single case with spectacular visual improvement from 20/100 to 20/25 [49].

IGS was also treated by adalimumab (Humira). No significant improvement after such therapy was achieved in a small case series of five eyes [50].

4. Discussion

The excellent results of modern cataract surgery set patient expectations very high, and persistent CME after uneventful cataract surgery may significantly affect patient outcomes and satisfaction [51]. Irvine–Gass syndrome is a common complication of uneventful cataract surgery, which resolves spontaneously in most cases but may persist, causing visual deterioration and patient dissatisfaction [4,6,7]. As has been emphasized in many previous reviews and studies, no homogenous recommendations for the treatment of IVG exist [52–55]. The lack of randomized controlled trials assessing the effectiveness of available therapeutic modalities results in many different approaches, often based on individual judgment and clinical experience but not hard evidence. Our analysis focused on the papers published in this century, as this is the time when intravitreal treatments such as anti-VEGF or intravitreal corticosteroids were introduced and revolutionized the management of various ophthalmic diseases. Therefore, we sought to compare conservative treatments to those modern therapeutic modalities.

Presented studies published since 2000^t in general show favorable results of the treatment of IGS with topical NSAIDs alone or in combination with periocular or intravitreal steroids as well as intravitreal anti-VEGF agents. Those treatments should be considered, weighing both the potential for improving BCVA and the invasive character of the treatment and the possibility of complications.

As IGS resolves spontaneously in most cases, that possibility must be considered before administering invasive therapy. Therefore, the timing of the application of different forms of treatment should be carefully considered with non-invasive therapies used as the first line (e.g., topical treatment) and invasive procedures (e.g., intraocular injections) usually reserved for non-responsive cases.

NSAIDs administered topically such as via eye drops are FDA-approved drugs for use as anti-inflammatory, antipyretic, and analgesic agents. Their main mechanism of action is the inhibition of the enzyme cyclooxygenase (COX). Cyclooxygenase is required to convert arachidonic acid into thromboxanes, prostaglandins, and prostacyclin. Prostaglandins play an important role in vasodilatation [56]. The use of NSAIDs in the postoperative management of patients undergoing cataract surgery has become a standard of care [57,58]. Routine use of anti-inflammatory eye drops following cataract surgery is highly effective in reducing post-surgical inflammation and the incidence of CME [59]; however, their role in the treatment of CME has not been studied widely. Topical NSAIDs remain a first-line therapy of IGS, and although their use has shown to be beneficial in several studies, they have shown no clear effect in other studies [58]. Our search revealed only a few modern studies that analyze the effects of NSAID in the treatment of IGS, none of which is an RCT. One older study showed significant visual and morphological improvements after administration of topical NSAID in acute cases, which are usually defined as lasting less than 3 months [18]. However, most recent studies show only moderate improvement after treatment of IGS with only topical NSAID [12,13].

Functional and morphological results are reported to be better after intravitreal dexamethasone [13]. Adding the effect of nepafenac was reported in one study that analyzed the combination of IVB and NSAID [16]. NSAIDs are also used in combined therapy with topical corticosteroids or oral CAIs, but available data on the combined treatment of CME are very limited. Nevertheless, the off-label use of acetazolamide, a carbonic anhydrase inhibitor, in IGS is a common practice as a first- or second-line therapy. Acetazolamide increases the retinal pigment epithelium pump function by inhibiting carbonic anhydrase and is thought to decrease intraretinal fluid [11,60]. Dosage varies among studies from 250 mg once a day to TID. Many authors state that the combination of oral acetazolamide with topical NSAIDs is shown to be highly effective [20,61,62]. Our search revealed only two papers analyzing the additional effect of CAI compared to NSAID-only treatment of IGS, both on relatively small samples (14–15 eyes). Both papers favor the use of CAI in combination therapy for IGS; however, such limited data make it impossible to build strong recommendations for the use of this treatment regimen.

Corticosteroids remain a viable therapeutic option in the treatment of CME, including IGS. Corticosteroids block the release of arachidonic acid, impact the production of interleukins and VEGF, and interrupt the inflammatory cascade. Several routes of administration, such as topical, periocular, and intravitreal, are available. At the same time, current data on a combination treatment of topical NSAID with topical corticosteroids are scarce and not convincing [21,22]. A conclusion on the beneficial effect of the addition of topical corticosteroids to the treatment of IGS cannot be made based on available research. Nevertheless, topical corticosteroids are widely used in the treatment of Irvine–Gass syndrome, usually in combination with topical NSAIDs and oral CAIs. An accurate assessment of the role of topical corticosteroids alone in the treatment of IGS is not currently possible.

Periocular or intravitreal corticosteroids serve as an option in refractory cases of IGS [63]. Sub-tenon or retrobulbar injections of corticosteroids had been used widely for persistent CME before the advent of an officially registered intravitreal dexamethasone implant (OZURDEX®). Early in 1997, Thach and his group showed VA improvement after 12 repeated corticosteroid injections in a series of 31 patients with chronic CME [64]. Our search revealed three recent studies (2018–2021) that showed significant visual improvement after STT in refractory cases of IGS. STT remains a cost-effective therapy, and its application sub-tenon does not bear the risk of intraocular inflammation possible after intravitreal application. A recent study by Kuley did not show an advantage of intravitreal versus sub-tenon administration of triamcinolone [23]. It must be emphasized, though, that the use of triamcinolone acetonide remains off-label. Intravitreal corticosteroids have consequently been used for chronic or refractory cases, lasting longer than 3 months, with significant letter gains and minor adverse effects [31–35]. Before the dexamethasone implant was introduced, triamcinolone acetonide was tested in a few larger and smaller studies, proving its efficacy in improving macular morphology and function in IGS [33,35,65–67]. Later studies show significant improvements after IVD administration without serious side effects [27,29–32,34]. The most recent large retrospective study from 2020 highlighted the benefits of early intervention and reported significantly larger visual gains when IVD was administered within 4 weeks of diagnosis [27]. This approach is not a common practice due to the invasive character of the procedure and the possibility of effective treatment with only topical NSAIDs. Further comparative studies are needed to support the results of that paper.

Vascular endothelial growth factors play central roles in the regulation of angiogenesis and lymphangiogenesis and they regulate endothelial cell proliferation, migration, vascular permeability, secretion, and other endothelial functions. The revolutionary role of anti-VEGF in treating ophthalmic conditions such as neovascularization and macular edema due to DME or ME in RVO was a milestone. The VEGF family plays a major role in angiogenesis, inflammation, and capillary permeability; thus, its potential in treating CME was studied. However, the role of anti-VEGF treatment in CME remains unclear. Anti-VEGF injections remain an alternative in unresponsive cases, but their use in IGS requires further randomized research. Our search revealed a few quality studies that show significant improvements after the use of anti-VEGF medication in IGS, but RCTs are missing. Despite that, clinical practice and the universality of that procedure make it a solid treatment modality in refractory IGS.

Non-damaging laser therapy, such as SML, remains an interesting therapeutic option. To date, just a few papers report its efficacy in IGS. Considering its non-damaging character, lack of side effects, and low cost, it may be considered as an alternative to more invasive treatment modalities. Further studies are needed to provide treatment guidelines for SML.

Practical Considerations and Conclusions

This review aimed to provide a basis for modern recommendations for treating pseudophakic macular edema or Irvine–Gass syndrome. The available published material does not provide convincing data to build such guidelines. Therefore, theoretical background, clinical experience, and safety of the procedure must determine the choice of treatment in this clinical entity. Common practice is to start therapy with a topical NSAID, which is a simple and non-invasive treatment modality. This approach is supported by epidemiological and clinical research that provides data on the possibility of spontaneous resolution of CME and improvement after topical therapy [68]. Larger clinical trials have not shown that using a combination of topical NSAID and topical corticosteroids and/or oral CAI is superior to topical NSAID alone.

What remains unclear is the timing of application of invasive therapies—periocular or intravitreal injections—once topical treatment is not effective. Refractory pseudophakic macular edema is not precisely defined according to its duration, but usually authors employ periocular or intravitreal treatment in cases lasting longer than three months. The efficacy and safety of intravitreal or periocular injections with corticosteroids or anti-VEGF agents have been confirmed in many studies. Still, its invasive nature and rare but potentially serious complications must be considered. Patients who resist intravitreal or periocular treatment might be offered therapy with subthreshold micropulse laser. Recent publications on the use of SML show promise. Low complication rates, cost-effectiveness, and repeatability are clear advantages of this treatment modality.

Our search revealed publications that show possible options for the treatment of IGS. Methodology and randomization in presented trials may be discussed; what remains as their common feature is the visual deficit reported in most cases of longstanding CME, even after successful treatment. Therefore, in view of results of a recent large study from Sharma et al. [27] that proves better functional and morphological results with early application of intravitreal steroids, that therapeutic option for short-standing pseudophakic CME should be examined with care in future research.

Author Contributions: Conceptualization: M.O. and M.G.; Methodology: M.G., Investigation: M.O. and M.G., writing: M.O. and M.G., supervision: M.G. All authors have read and agreed to the published version of the manuscript.

Funding: This research received no external funding.

Institutional Review Board Statement: Not applicable.

Informed Consent Statement: Not applicable.

Data Availability Statement: Not applicable.

Conflicts of Interest: The authors declare no conflict of interest.

References

1. Grzybowski, A.; Sikorski, B.L.; Ascano, F.J.; Huerva, V. Pseudophakic cystoid macular edema. *Clin. Interv. Aging* **2016**, *11*, 1221–1229. [CrossRef] [PubMed]
2. Irvine, S.R. A newly defined vitreous syndrome following cataract surgery. *Am. J. Ophthalmol.* **1953**, *36*, 599–619. [CrossRef]
3. Gass, J.D.; Norton, E.W. Cystoid macular edema and papilledema following cataract extraction. A fluorescein fundoscopic and angiographic study. *Arch. Ophthalmol.* **1966**, *76*, 646–661. [CrossRef] [PubMed]
4. Henderson, B.A.; Kim, J.Y.; Ament, C.S.; Ferrufino-Ponce, Z.K.; Grabowska, A.; Cremers, S.L. Clinical pseudophakic cystoid macular edema. Risk factors for development and duration after treatment. *J. Cataract Refract. Surg.* **2007**, *33*, 1550–1558. [CrossRef] [PubMed]

5. Hunter, A.A.; Modjtahedi, S.P.; Long, K.; Zawadzki, R.; Chin, E.K.; Caspar, J.J.; Morse, L.S.; Telander, D.G. Improving visual outcomes by preserving outer retina morphology in eyes with resolved pseudophakic cystoid macular edema. *J. Cataract Refract. Surg.* **2014**, *40*, 626–631. [CrossRef]
6. Flach, A.J. The incidence, pathogenesis and treatment of cystoid macular edema following cataract surgery. *Trans. Am. Ophthalmol. Soc.* **1998**, *96*, 557–634.
7. Perente, I.; Utine, C.A.; Ozturker, C.; Cakir, M.; Kaya, V.; Eren, H.; Kapran, Z.; Yilmaz, O.F. Evaluation of macular changes after uncomplicated phacoemulsification surgery by optical coherence tomography. *Curr. Eye Res.* **2007**, *32*, 241–247. [CrossRef]
8. Ursell, P.G.; Spalton, D.J.; Whitcup, S.M.; Nussenblatt, R.B. Cystoid macular edema after phacoemulsification: Relationship to blood-aqueous barrier damage and visual acuity. *J. Cataract Refract. Surg.* **1999**, *25*, 1492–1497. [CrossRef]
9. Shelsta, H.N.; Jampol, L.M. Pharmacologic therapy of pseudophakic cystoid macular edema: 2010 update. *Retina* **2011**, *31*, 4–12. [CrossRef] [PubMed]
10. Smith, R.T.; Campbell, C.J.; Koester, C.J.; Trokel, S.; Anderson, A. The barrier function in extracapsular cataract surgery. *Ophthalmology* **1990**, *97*. [CrossRef]
11. Benitah, N.R.; Arroyo, J.G. Pseudophakic cystoid macular edema. *Int. Ophthalmol. Clin.* **2010**, *50*, 139–153. [CrossRef]
12. Giarmoukakis, A.K.; Blazaki, S.V.; Bontzos, G.C.; Plaka, A.D.; Seliniotakis, K.N.; Ioannidi, L.D.; Tsilimbaris, M.K. Efficacy of topical nepafenac 0.3% in the management of postoperative cystoid macular edema. *Ther. Clin. Risk Manag.* **2020**, *16*, 1067–1074. [CrossRef]
13. Guclu, H.; Gurlu, V.P. Comparison of topical nepafenac 0.1% with intravitreal dexamethasone implant for the treatment of Irvine-Gass syndrome. *Int. J. Ophthalmol.* **2019**, *12*, 258–267. [CrossRef] [PubMed]
14. Sengupta, S.; Vasavada, D.; Pan, U.; Sindal, M. Factors predicting response of pseudophakic cystoid macular edema to topical steroids and nepafenac. *Indian J. Ophthalmol.* **2018**, *66*, 827–830. [CrossRef] [PubMed]
15. Yüksel, B.; Uzunel, U.D.; Kerci, S.G.; Sağban, L.; Kusbeci, T.; Örsel, T. Comparison of subtenon triamcinolone acetonide injection with topical nepafenac for the treatment of pseudophakic cystoid macular edema. *Ocul. Immunol. Inflamm.* **2016**, *25*, 513–519. [CrossRef]
16. Warren, K.A.; Bahrani, H.; Fox, J.E. NSAIDs in combination therapy for the treatment of chronic pseudophakic cystoid macular edema. *Retina* **2010**, *30*, 260–266. [CrossRef] [PubMed]
17. Hariprasad, S.M.; Akduman, L.; Clever, J.A.; Ober, M.; Recchia, F.M.; Mieler, W.F. Treatment of cystoid macular edema with the new-generation NSAID nepafenac 0.1%. *Clin. Ophthalmol.* **2009**, *3*, 147–154. [CrossRef]
18. Rho, D.S. Treatment of acute pseudophakic cystoid macular edema: Diclofenac versus ketorolac. *J. Cataract Refract. Surg.* **2003**, *29*, 2378–2384. [CrossRef]
19. Curković, T.; Vukojević, N.; Bućan, K. Treatment of pseudophakic cystoid macular oedema. *Coll. Antropol.* **2005**, 103–105.
20. Catier, A.; Tadayoni, R.; Massin, P.; Gaudric, A. Intérêt de l'acétazolamide associé aux anti-inflammatoires dans le traitement de l'oedème maculaire postopératoire (Advantages of acetazolamide associated with anti-inflammatory medications in postoperative treatment of macular edema). *J. Fr. Ophthalmol.* **2005**, *28*, 1027–1031. [CrossRef]
21. Heier, J.S.; Topping, T.M.; Baumann, W.; Dirks, M.S.; Chern, S. Ketorolac versus prednisolone versus combination therapy in the treatment of acute pseudophakic cystoid macular edema. *Ophthalmology* **2000**, *107*, 2034–2038. [CrossRef]
22. Singal, N.; Hopkins, J. Pseudophakic cystoid macular edema: Ketorolac alone vs. ketorolac plus prednisolone. *Can. J. Ophthalmol.* **2004**, *39*, 245–250. [CrossRef]
23. Kuley, B.; Storey, P.P.; Wibbelsman, T.D.; Pancholy, M.; Zhang, Q.; Sharpe, J.; Bello, N.; Obeid, A.; Regillo, C.; Kaiser, R.S.; et al. Resolution of pseudophakic cystoid macular edema: 2 mg intravitreal triamcinolone acetonide versus 40 mg posterior sub-tenon triamcinolone acetonide. *Curr. Eye Res.* **2021**, 1–7. [CrossRef]
24. Erden, B.; Çakır, A.; Aslan, A.C.; Bölükbaşı, S.; Elçioğlu, M.N. The efficacy of posterior subtenon triamcinolone acetonide injection in treatment of irvine-gass syndrome. *Ocul. Immunol. Inflamm.* **2019**, *27*, 1235–1241. [CrossRef]
25. Tsai, M.-J.; Yang, C.-M.; Hsieh, Y.-T. Posterior subtenon injection of triamcinolone acetonide for pseudophakic cystoid macular oedema. *Acta Ophthalmol.* **2016**, *96*, e891–e893. [CrossRef]
26. Benhamou, N.; Massin, P.; Haouchine, B.; Audren, F.; Tadayoni, R.; Gaudric, A. Intravitreal triamcinolone for refractory pseudophakic macular edema. *Am. J. Ophthalmol.* **2003**, *135*, 246–249. [CrossRef]
27. Sharma, A.; Bandello, F.; Loewenstein, A.; Kuppermann, B.D.; Lanzetta, P.; Zur, D.; Hilely, A.; Iglicki, M.; Veritti, D.; Wang, A.; et al. Current role of intravitreal injections in Irvine Gass syndrome-CRIIG study. *Int. Ophthalmol.* **2020**, *40*, 3067–3075. [CrossRef] [PubMed]
28. Marques, J.H.; Abreu, A.C.; Silva, N.; Meireles, A.; Pessoa, B.; Melo Beirão, J. Fluocinolone acetonide 0.19 mg implant in patients with cystoid macular edema due to Irvine-Gass syndrome. *Int. Med. Case Rep. J.* **2021**, *26*, 127–132. [CrossRef] [PubMed]
29. Altintas, A.G.K.; Ilhan, C. Intravitreal dexamethasone implantation in intravitreal bevacizumab treatment-resistant pseudophakic cystoid macular edema. *Korean J. Ophthalmol.* **2019**, *33*, 259–266. [CrossRef] [PubMed]
30. Bellocq, D.; Pierre-Kahn, V.; Matonti, F.; Burillon, C.; Voirin, N.; Dot, C.; Akesbi, J.; Milazzo, S.; Baillif, S.; Soler, V.; et al. Effectiveness and safety of dexamethasone implants for postsurgical macular oedema including Irvine–Gass syndrome: The EPISODIC-2 study. *Br. J. Ophthalmol.* **2016**, *101*, 333–341. [CrossRef] [PubMed]

31. Mayer, W.J.; Kurz, S.; Wolf, A.; Kook, D.; Kreutzer, T.; Kampik, A.; Priglinger, S.; Haritoglou, C. Dexamethasone implant as an effective treatment option for macular edema due to Irvine-Gass syndrome. *J. Cataract Refract. Surg.* **2015**, *41*, 1954–1961. [CrossRef] [PubMed]
32. Al Zamil, W.M. Short-term safety and efficacy of intravitreal 0.7-mg dexamethasone implants for pseudophakic cystoid macular edema. *Saudi J. Ophthalmol.* **2014**, *29*, 130–134. [CrossRef]
33. Sevim, M.; Sanisoglu, H.; Türkyılmaz, K. Intravitreal triamcinolone acetonide versus pars plana vitrectomy for pseudophakic cystoid macular edema. *Curr. Eye Res.* **2012**, *37*, 1165–1170. [CrossRef]
34. Williams, G.A.; Haller, J.A.; Kuppermann, B.D.; Blumenkranz, M.S.; Weinberg, D.V.; Chou, C.; Whitcup, S.M. Dexamethasone DDS phase II study group. Dexamethasone posterior-segment drug delivery system in the treatment of macular edema resulting from uveitis or Irvine-Gass syndrome. *Am. J. Ophthalmol.* **2009**, *147*, 1048–1054. [CrossRef]
35. Koutsandrea, C.; Moschos, M.M.; Brouzas, D.; Loukianou, E.; Apostolopoulos, M.; Moschos, M. Intraocular triamcinolone acetonide for pseudophakic cystoid macular edema: Optical coherence tomography and multifocal electroretinography study. *Retina* **2007**, *27*, 159–164. [CrossRef] [PubMed]
36. Lin, C.J.; Tsai, Y.Y. Use of aflibercept for the management of refractory pseudophakic macular edema in Irvine-Gass syndrome nad literature review. *Retin. Cases Brief. Rep.* **2018**, *12*, 59–62. [CrossRef]
37. Fenicia, V.; Balestrieri, M.; Perdicchi, A.; Enrici, M.M.; Fave, M.D.; Recupero, S.M. Intravitreal injection of dexamethasone implant and ranibizumab in cystoid macular edema in the course of Irvine-Gass syndrome. *Case Rep. Ophthalmol.* **2014**, *5*, 243–248. [CrossRef]
38. Akay, F.; Isik, M.U.; Akmaz, B. Comparison of intravitreal anti-vascular endothelial growth factor agents and treatment results in Irvine-Gass syndrome. *Int. J. Ophthalmol.* **2020**, *13*, 1586–1591. [CrossRef]
39. Staurenghi, G.; Lai, T.Y.Y.; Mitchell, P.; Wolf, S.; Wenzel, A.; Li, J.; Bhaumik, A.; Hykin, P.G.; PROMETHEUS Study Group. Efficacy and safety of ranibizumab 0.5 mg for the treatment of macular edema resulting from uncommon causes: Twelve-month findings from prometheus. *Ophthalmology* **2018**, *125*, 850–862. [CrossRef] [PubMed]
40. Arevalo, J.F.; Maia, M.; Garcia-Amaris, R.A.; Roca, J.A.; Sanchez, J.G.; Berrocal, M.H.; Wu, L. Intravitreal bevacizumab for refractory pseudophakic cystoid macular edema: The Pan-American collaborative retina study group results. *Ophthalmology* **2009**, *116*, 1481.e1–1487.e1. [CrossRef]
41. Barone, A.; Russo, V.; Prascina, F.; Noci, N.D. Short-term safety and efficacy of intravitreal bevacizumab for pseudophakic macular edema. *Retina* **2009**, *29*, 33–37. [CrossRef]
42. Spitzer, M.S.; Ziemssen, F.; Yoeruek, E.; Petermeier, K.; Aisenbrey, S.; Szurman, P. Efficacy of intravitreal bevacizumab in treating postoperative pseudophakic cystoid macular edema. *J. Cataract Refract. Surg.* **2008**, *34*, 70–75. [CrossRef]
43. Arevalo, J.F.; Garcia-Amaris, R.A.; Roca, J.A.; Sanchez, J.G.; Wu, L.; Berrocal, M.H.; Maia, M. Primary intravitreal bevacizumab for the management of pseudophakic cystoid macular edema: Pilot study of the Pan-American collaborative retina study Group. *J. Cataract Refract. Surg.* **2007**, *339120*, 2098–3105. [CrossRef] [PubMed]
44. Gawęcki, M. Micropulse laser treatment of retinal diseases. *J. Clin. Med.* **2019**, *8*, 242. [CrossRef]
45. Gawęcki, M.; Jaszczuk-Maciejewska, A.; Jurska-Jaśko, A.; Kneba, M.; Grzybowski, A. Transfoveal micropulse laser treatment of central serous chorioretinopathy within six months of disease onset. *J. Clin. Med.* **2019**, *8*, 1398. [CrossRef] [PubMed]
46. Verdina, T.; D'Aloisio, R.; Lazzerini, A.; Ferrari, C.; Valerio, E.; Mastropasqua, R.; Cavallini, G.M. The role of subthreshold micropulse yellow laser as an alternative option for the treatment of refractory postoperative cystoid macular edema. *J. Clin. Med.* **2020**, *9*, 1066. [CrossRef]
47. Lardenoye, C.W.; van Schooneveld, M.J.; Frits Treffers, W.; Rothova, A. Grid laser photocoagulation for macular oedema in uveitis or the Irvine-Gass syndrome. *Br. J. Ophthalmol.* **1998**, *82*, 1013–1016. [CrossRef]
48. Deuter, C.M.E.; Gelisken, F.; Stübiger, N.; Zierhut, M.; Doycheva, D. Successful treatment of chronic pseudophakic macular edema (Irvine-Gass syndrome) with interferon alpha: A report of three cases. *Ocul. Immunol. Inflamm.* **2011**, *19*, 216–218. [CrossRef] [PubMed]
49. Maleki, A.; Aghaei, H.; Lee, S. Topical interferon alpha 2b in the treatment of refractory pseudophakic cystoid macular edema. *Am. J. Ophthalmol. Case Rep.* **2018**, *10*, 203–205. [CrossRef]
50. Farvardin, M.; Namvar, E.; Sanie-Jahromi, F.; Johari, M.K. The effects of intravitreal adalimumab injection on pseudophakic macular edema. *BMC Res. Notes* **2020**, *13*, 1–4. [CrossRef]
51. Gawęcki, M.; Grzybowski, A. Diplopia as the complication of cataract surgery. *J. Ophthalmol.* **2016**, *2016*, 1–6. [CrossRef]
52. Tsangaridou, M.-A.; Grzybowski, A.; Gundlach, E.; Pleyer, U. Controversies in NSAIDs use in cataract surgery. *Curr. Pharm. Des.* **2015**, *21*, 4707–4717. [CrossRef]
53. Grzybowski, A.; Kanclerz, P. Controversies on the use of nonsteroidal antiinflammatory drugs and steroids in pseudophakic cystoid macular edema prophylaxis. *J. Cataract Refract. Surg.* **2019**, *45*, 1848. [PubMed]
54. Guo, S.; Patel, S.; Baumrind, B.; Johnson, K.; Levinsohn, D.; Marcus, E.; Tannen, B.; Roy, M.; Bhagat, N.; Zarbin, M. Management of pseudophakic cystoid macular edema. *Surv. Ophthalmol.* **2015**, *60*, 123–137. [CrossRef]
55. Yonekawa, Y.; Kim, I.K. Pseudophakic cystoid macular edema. *Curr. Opin. Ophthalmol.* **2012**, *23*, 26–32. [CrossRef] [PubMed]
56. Vane, J.R. Inhibition of prostaglandin synthesis as a mechanism of action for aspirin-like drugs. *Nat. New Biol.* **1971**, *231*, 232–235. [CrossRef] [PubMed]

57. Brandsdorfer, A.; Patel, S.H.; Chuck, R.S. The role of perioperative nonsteroidal anti-inflammatory drugs use in cataract surgery. *Curr. Opin. Ophthalmol.* **2019**, *30*, 44–49. [CrossRef] [PubMed]
58. Lim, B.X.; Lim, C.H.; Lim, D.K.; Evans, J.R.; Bunce, C.; Wormald, R. Prophylactic non-steroidal anti-inflammatory drugs for the prevention of macular oedema after cataract surgery. *Cochrane Database Syst. Rev.* **2016**. [CrossRef] [PubMed]
59. Rossetti, L.; Chaudhuri, J.; Dickersin, K. Medical prophylaxis and treatment of cystoid macular edema after cataract surgery: The results of a meta-analysis. *Ophthalmology* **1998**, *105*, 397–405. [CrossRef]
60. Marmor, M.F.; Maack, T. Enhancement of retinal adhesion and sub- retinal fluid resorption by acetazolamide. *Invest. Ophthalmol. Vis. Sci.* **1982**, *23*, 121–124.
61. Cox, S.N.; Hay, E.; Bird, A.C. Treatment of chronic macular edema with acetazolamide. *Arch. Ophthalmol.* **1988**, *106*, 1190–1195. [CrossRef]
62. Weene, L. Cystoid macular edema after scleral buckling responsive to acetazolamide. *Ann. Ophthalmol.* **1992**, *24*.
63. Zur, D.; Loewenstein, A. Postsurgical cystoid macular edema. *Dev. Ophthalmol.* **2017**, *58*, 178–190. [CrossRef] [PubMed]
64. Thach, A.B.; Dugel, P.U.; Flindall, R.J.; Sipperley, J.O.; Sneed, S.R. A Comparison of retrobulbar versus sub-tenon's corticosteroid therapy for cystoid macular edema refractory to topical medications. *Ophthalmology* **1997**, *104*, 2003–2008. [CrossRef]
65. Boscia, F.; Furino, C.; Dammacco, R.; Ferreri, P.; Sborgia, L. Intravitreal triamcinolone acetonide in refractory pseudophakic cystoid macular edema: Functional and anatomic results. *Eur. J. Ophthalmol.* **2005**, *15*, 89–95. [CrossRef] [PubMed]
66. Jonas, J.B.; Kreissig, I.; Degenring, R.F. Intravitreal triamcinolone acetonide for pseudophakic cystoid macular edema. *Am. J. Ophthalmol.* **2003**, *136*, 384–386. [CrossRef]
67. Conway, M.D.; Canakis, C.; Livir-Rallatos, C.; Peyman, G.A. Intravitreal triamcinolone acetonide for refractory chronic pseudophakic cystoid macular edema. *J. Cataract Refract. Surg.* **2003**, *29*, 27–33. [CrossRef]
68. Zur, D.; Fischer, N.; Tufail, A.; Monés, J.; Loewenstein, A. Postsurgical cystoid macular edema. *Eur. J. Ophthalmol.* **2011**, *21*, 62–68. [CrossRef]

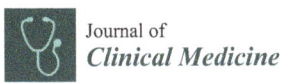

Article

Imbalance in the Levels of Angiogenic Factors in Patients with Acute and Chronic Central Serous Chorioretinopathy

Izabella Karska-Basta [1,*], Weronika Pociej-Marciak [1], Michał Chrząszcz [1], Agnieszka Kubicka-Trząska [1], Magdalena Dębicka-Kumela [1], Maciej Gawęcki [2], Bożena Romanowska-Dixon [1] and Marek Sanak [3]

[1] Department of Ophthalmology, Faculty of Medicine, Clinic of Ophthalmology and Ocular Oncology, Jagiellonian University Medical College, 31-070 Krakow, Poland; weronika.pociej-marciak@uj.edu.pl (W.P.-M.); m.a.chrzaszcz@gmail.com (M.C.); agnieszka.kubicka-trzaska@uj.edu.pl (A.K.-T.); magdalena.debicka-kumela@uj.edu.pl (M.D.-K.); romanowskadixonbozena1@gmail.com (B.R.-D.)

[2] Dobry Wzrok Ophthalmological Clinic, 80-402 Gdansk, Poland; maciej@gawecki.com

[3] Molecular Biology and Clinical Genetics Unit, Department of Internal Medicine, Jagiellonian University Medical College Faculty of Medicine, 31-066 Krakow, Poland; marek.sanak@uj.edu.pl

* Correspondence: izabasta@gmail.com

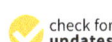

Citation: Karska-Basta, I.; Pociej-Marciak, W.; Chrząszcz, M.; Kubicka-Trząska, A.; Dębicka-Kumela, M.; Gawęcki, M.; Romanowska-Dixon, B.; Sanak, M. Imbalance in the Levels of Angiogenic Factors in Patients with Acute and Chronic Central Serous Chorioretinopathy. *J. Clin. Med.* **2021**, *10*, 1087. https://doi.org/10.3390/jcm10051087

Academic Editor: Fumi Gomi

Received: 21 January 2021
Accepted: 26 February 2021
Published: 5 March 2021

Publisher's Note: MDPI stays neutral with regard to jurisdictional claims in published maps and institutional affiliations.

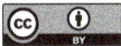

Copyright: © 2021 by the authors. Licensee MDPI, Basel, Switzerland. This article is an open access article distributed under the terms and conditions of the Creative Commons Attribution (CC BY) license (https://creativecommons.org/licenses/by/4.0/).

Abstract: Background: The pathogenesis of central serous chorioretinopathy (CSC) remains a subject of intensive research. We aimed to determine correlations between plasma levels of selected angiogenic factors and different forms of CSC. Methods: Eighty patients were enrolled in the study including 30 with a chronic form of CSC, 30 with acute CSC, and 20 controls. Presence of active CSC was determined by fluorescein angiography (FA), indocyanine green angiography (ICGA), and swept-source optical coherence tomography (SS-OCT). Plasma concentrations of angiopoietin-1, endostatin, fibroblast growth factor, placental growth factor (PlGF), platelet-derived growth factor (PDGF-AA), thrombospondin-2, vascular endothelial growth factor (VEGF), VEGF-D, and pigment epithelium–derived factor were measured, and the results were compared between groups. Additionally, mean choroidal thickness (CT) was measured in all patients. Results: Levels of angiopoietin-1 ($p = 0.008$), PlGF ($p = 0.045$), and PDGF-AA ($p = 0.033$) differed significantly between the three groups. Compared with the controls, VEGF ($p = 0.024$), PlGF ($p = 0.013$), and PDGF-AA ($p = 0.012$) were downregulated in the whole CSC group, specifically PDGF-AA ($p = 0.002$) in acute CSC and angiopoietin-1 ($p = 0.007$) in chronic CSC. An inverse correlation between mean CT and VEGF levels was noted in CSC patients ($rho = -0.27$, $p = 0.044$). Conclusions: Downregulated angiopoietin-1, VEGF, PDGF-AA, and PlGF levels may highlight the previously unknown role of the imbalanced levels of proangiogenic and antiangiogenic factors in the pathogenesis of CSC. Moreover, downregulated VEGF levels may suggest that choroidal neovascularization in CSC is associated with arteriogenesis rather than angiogenesis.

Keywords: angiogenesis; angiopoietin-1; central serous chorioretinopathy; proangiogenic factors

1. Introduction

Central serous chorioretinopathy (CSC) is a common disease that belongs to the pachychoroid-related disorders, characterized by serous retinal detachment, which is associated with a local leakage from the thicker choroid through impaired retinal pigment epithelium (RPE) [1]. For a long time, a simple classification of CSC into acute and chronic forms has been used; however, it was based solely on the duration of serous neurosensory retinal detachment [2]. Nowadays, as new pathogenic concepts of CSC emerge and modern multimodal imaging becomes available, various new classifications are being developed, but so far, none of them has fully reflected the complexity of this clinical entity [3,4]. Daruich et al. classified CSC as acute, non-resolving, recurrent, chronic, or inactive, which more precisely refers to the course of the disease [5].

As the pathogenesis and pathophysiology of CSC have not been fully explained, the available treatment modalities are suboptimal, especially in long-standing cases [2,6]. Growing evidence indicates that the pathomechanism of CSC is associated with dysfunction of the thickened choroid (an important risk factor), with subsequent impairment of the RPE [1,7]. Some authors have also postulated that downregulation of the cell–cell adhesion molecules in the vascular endothelium could increase the permeability of choroidal vessels, causing fluid leakage under the neurosensory retina [8,9]. In the present study, we attempted to find an association between these phenomena in CSC and the levels of proangiogenic and antiangiogenic factors in human plasma.

Although the role of elevated levels of vascular endothelial growth factor (VEGF) and other cytokines in the pathogenesis of the pachychoroid disease has been speculated on in some papers, they more often referred to other forms of this disease entity than CSC [10,11]. Recent studies suggested that eyes with CSC may be at higher risk of age-related macular degeneration (AMD) or one of its subtypes (polypoidal choroidal vasculopathy or pachychoroid neovasculopathy), or that the development of CSC and AMD/polypoidal choroidal vasculopathy may share a common background [12–14]. Data on systemic changes in the expression of proangiogenic and antiangiogenic factors and their role in choroidal vascular homeostasis associated with CSC are scarce. Apart from our previous research, we identified only one report evaluating the plasma level of VEGF in patients with CSC [15,16].

It is well-known that CSC may be complicated by choroidal neovascularization (CNV), a typical feature for neovascular AMD (nAMD). The prevalence of this complication was reported to range from 15.6% to 25% [16,17]. Extensive research of AMD included the levels of proangiogenic factors [18–20]. Impaired expression of antiangiogenic factors was shown to play an important role in the development of CNV in the course of nAMD [21]. By analogy, some of these etiological factors typical for nAMD could also be involved in the course of different forms of pachychoroid disease such as CSC. Interestingly, whereas acute exposure to some angiogenic factors such as VEGF results in fast but self-limited hyperpermeability of normal vessels, chronic exposure leads to profound changes in venular function and structure, which results in its chronic hyperpermeability and pathological vessel formation [22]. Angiogenesis and arteriogenesis play a crucial role in tissue development, repair, and regeneration, but also in ocular pathology [23]. Both processes depend on the intricate balance of angiogenic and inflammatory factors [24,25].

To our knowledge, no studies have reported alterations in the levels of circulating angiogenic factors in patients with CSC, which is not an angiogenic condition in itself, but since it is a pachychoroid disease, its phenotype is characterized by attenuation of the choriocapillaris overlying dilated choroidal veins [7]. The purpose of our study was to highlight the previously unknown role of the imbalanced levels of proangiogenic and antiangiogenic factors in CSC. Additionally, our findings may support the search for new therapeutic strategies in CSC and provide new targets for development in the field.

2. Materials and Methods

This case-control study included 60 white adult patients (11 women and 49 men) diagnosed with CSC in the Department of Ophthalmology and Ocular Oncology in Kraków, Poland, between November 2017 and June 2018. The control group comprised 20 healthy volunteers from the University Hospital in Kraków, who were matched for sex, age, smoking status, and hypertension. The diagnosis of CSC was based on characteristic findings of indirect ophthalmoscopy, fluorescein angiography (FA), indocyanine green angiography (ICGA, SPECTRALIS, Heidelberg Engineering, Heidelberg, Germany), and SS-OCT (DRI OCT Atlantis, Topcon, Japan). Ocular exclusion criteria were as follows: nAMD, uveitis, diabetic retinopathy, vasculitis, polypoidal choroidal vasculopathy, neovascular glaucoma, anti-VEGF treatment, and other diseases causing macular exudation. Systemic exclusion criteria included any malignancy, acute illness, rheumatoid arthritis, psoriasis, renal or hepatic dysfunction, acute myocardial infarction or stroke within the preceding six months, and corticosteroid treatment. The study was approved by Jagiellonian University Bioethical Committee (Approval No. 122.6120.266.2016), and all patients and controls provided written informed consent to participate in the study.

2.1. Clinical Examination

The measurement of best-corrected visual acuity, indirect ophthalmoscopy of the fundus, and SS-OCT were performed in all groups, whereas FA and ICGA were performed only in the CSC group. Central serous chorioretinopathy was classified as acute when symptoms and clinical signs lasted less than six months, whereas chronic CSC was diagnosed when symptoms lasted six months or longer.

The diagnosis of CSC was based on the SS-OCT, FA, and ICGA findings. For SS-OCT, the criteria included current or previous pigment epithelium detachment and/or serous retinal detachment as well as increased CT. On FA, symptoms characteristic for CSC were sought such as focal or multispot dye leakage, dye pooling, or widespread areas of granular hyperfluorescence. Finally, for ICGA, remarkable findings included areas of persistent hyperpermeability during the early and middle phases as well as central hyperfluorescence during the late phase.

Choroidal thickness was assessed using the method previously described by Branchini et al. [26]. Mean CT was considered as the average of the measurements from three points, which were localized beneath the fovea as well as 750 µm temporally and 750 µm nasally from the fovea. The measurements were done by two experienced ophthalmologists (AKT and IKB).

2.2. Sample Collection

Blood was drawn from the antecubital vein into BD Vacutainer (BD Life Sciences, Franklin Lakes, NJ, USA) from all participants. Tubes contained (EDTA) as an anticoagulant for plasma preparation. The plasma levels of 10 different angiogenic proteins were measured using the Human Angiogenesis A Premixed Mag Luminex Performance Assay (FCSTM02-10, R&D Systems, Minneapolis, MI, USA). This multiplex immunoassay contains premixed fluorogenic beads with monoclonal antibodies against angiogenin, angiopoietin-1, endostatin, FGF-acidic, FGF-basic, PlGF, PDGF-AA, thrombospondin-2, VEGF, and VEGF-D. The measurements were done according to the manufacturer's protocol using 1:4 diluted plasma and the xMAP analyzer (Luminex Corporation, Austin, TX, USA). Bead-trapped cytokines were detected by biotin-streptavidin sandwich immunocomplex fluorescence. The results were calculated using 7-point standard curves and proprietary software, Milliplex Analyst Version 5.1 (Merck, Darmstadt, Germany). The plasma levels of angiogenin exceeded the highest concentration of the standard curve calibrator (29,900 pg/mL) in 94% of the samples; therefore, they were not included in further analysis.

2.3. Statistical Analysis

Qualitative data were presented as counts and percentages. Quantitative data were shown as means and standard deviations (SD) for normally distributed variables and as medians (Me) and interquartile ranges (IQRs) otherwise. The normality of quantitative variables was tested using the Kolmogorov–Smirnov test. Intergroup comparisons of qualitative variables were made using the Pearson 2 test; this test was used when expected frequencies in more than 80% of cells were higher than five; and the Fisher–Freeman–Halton test was used otherwise. Intergroup comparisons of quantitative variables were made using the 1-way analysis of variance (ANOVA) for normally distributed variables and the Kruskal–Wallis test for variables with nonnormal distribution. When the comparison of the three groups yielded a significant p value, a pairwise comparison with Bonferroni correction was used. For FGF-acidic, the ANOVA was used after removing one outlier case present in the acute-CSC group. The CSC (both chronic and acute) and control groups were compared using the t-test or Mann–Whitney test, as appropriate. The results of the comparison were presented graphically with a box plot, where the line inside the box represents a median; the lower and upper sides of the box represent the lower and upper quartiles, respectively; the horizontal lines connected to the box with vertical lines represent cases distant up to 1.5 of the IQR from the respective quartiles; circles represent cases distant from 1.5 to 3 IQRs from the respective quartile; and asterisks represent cases distant by more than 3 IQRs from the respective quartile. The strength of the relationship between quantitative variables was estimated using the Spearman rank correlation coefficient. A p value of less than 0.05 was considered significant. The analysis was performed with IBM SPSS Statistics 24 for Windows statistical package.

3. Results

In the group with acute CSC ($n = 30$), 83.3% of patients were male compared with 80.0% in the group with chronic CSC ($n = 30$) and 55% in the control group ($n = 20$). The mean (SD) age was 42.7 (9.9) years for patients with acute CSC, 44.5 (6.1) years for those with chronic CSC, and 39.2 (7.4) years for the controls. The demographic and clinical characteristics of the groups are presented in Table 1. Patients with CSC and controls did not differ with regard to age, sex, smoking status, and the prevalence of systemic hypertension. Among the 11 women with CSC, three were after menopause and two used hormonal contraception. Angiotensin-converting enzyme inhibitors were used by four patients with acute CSC, two patients with chronic CSC, and three controls; β-blockers, by one patient with chronic CSC and one control; calcium channel blockers, by four patients with acute CSC and one patient with chronic CSC; diuretics, by six patients with acute CSC, five with chronic CSC, and one control. Finally, sartans were used by one patient with acute CSC and two patients with chronic CSC. Three patients with acute CSC did not use any antihypertensive treatment.

Table 1. Demographic and clinical characteristics of patients with acute and chronic central serous chorioretinopathy as well as controls.

Variable	Chronic CSC ($n = 30$)	Acute CSC ($n = 30$)	Controls ($n = 20$)	p Value
Male sex, n (%)	24 (80.0)	25 (83.3)	11 (55.0)	0.056 [1]
Age, y	44.5 (6.1)	42.7 (9.9)	39.2 (7.4)	0.078 [2]
Smoking (current, former), n (%)	8 (26.7)	7 (23.3)	7 (35.0)	0.658 [3]
Hypertension, n (%)	6 (20.0)	11 (36.7)	4 (20.0)	0.26 [4]
Hashimoto thyroiditis, n (%)	2 (6)	1 (3)	0 (0)	0.781
Helicobacter pylori infection, n (%)	6 (20)	0 (0)	0 (0)	0.007
Gout, n (%)	2 (6)	1 (3)	0 (0)	0.781
Ischemic heart disease, n (%)	1 (3)	1 (3)	0 (0)	1.000

[1] $\chi^2(2) = 5.778$; [2] $F(2,77) = 2.639$; [3] $\chi^2(2) = 0.836$; [4] $\chi^2(2) = 2.690$. Data were expressed as mean and standard deviation where the analysis of variance was used for comparisons unless specified as number (percentage) using the Pearson χ2 test or the Fisher–Freeman–Halton test as appropriate. A p value of less than 0.05 was considered significant. Abbreviations: CSC, central serous chorioretinopathy.

No significant differences were observed in the levels of the studied parameters between patients using at least one antihypertensive drug and those not receiving any antihypertensive medication: PEDF (Me = 94.99, Q1 = 60.99, Q3 = 198.66 and Me = 82.90, Q1 = 47.91, Q3 = 171.66, respectively, $p = 0.508$), FGF-basic (Me = 49.97, Q1 = 48.54, Q3 = 51.37 and Me = 48.54, Q1 = 46.60, Q3 = 51.36, respectively, $p = 0.234$), endostatin (Me = 20,098, Q1 = 16,908, Q3 = 22,640 and Me = 17,684, Q1 = 14,759, Q3 = 19,784, respectively, $p = 0.05$), FGF-acidic (Me = 129.91, Q1 = 125.39, Q3 = 134.43 and Me = 125.39, Q1 = 118.58, Q3 = 129.91, respectively, $p = 0.067$), PDGF-AA Me = 177.81, Q1 = 114.33, Q3 = 256.46 and Me = 191.2, Q1 = 137.72, Q3 = 252.15, respectively, $p = 0.557$), PlGF (Me = 3.24, Q1 = 2.9, Q3 = 4.48 and Me = 3.41, Q1 = 2.9, Q3 = 3.94, respectively, $p = 0.931$), VEGF-D (Me = 79.41, Q1 = 75.32, Q3 = 86.28 and Me = 78.05, Q1 = 72.61, Q3 = 83.52, respectively, $p = 0.182$), thrombospondin-2 (Me = 5534, Q1 = 4455, Q3 = 6725 and Me = 5321,

Q1 = 4113, Q3 = 6642, respectively, p = 0.553), angiopoetin-1 (Me = 2356, Q1 = 1129, Q3 = 3760 and Me = 2926, Q1 = 1819, Q3 = 3958, respectively, p = 0.224), and VEGF (Me = 12.5, Q1 = 5.2, Q3 = 20.5 and Me = 9.8, Q1 = 6.8, Q3 = 16.8, respectively, p = 0.968).

The baseline ophthalmological characteristics of patients and controls are presented in Table 2. The groups differed significantly in terms of best-corrected visual acuity and mean CT (Table 2).

Table 2. Ophthalmological characteristics of patients with acute and chronic central serous chorioretinopathy as well as controls.

Variable		Chronic CSC (n = 30)	Acute CSC (n = 30)	Controls (n = 20)	p Value
CT, μm		406.1 (88.1)	421.5 (85.3)	317.4 (61.4)	<0.001 [1]
Affected eye, n (%)	Right	10 (33.3)	14 (46.7)	-	0.225 [2]
	Left	12 (40)	13 (43.3)	-	
	Both	8 (26.7)	3 (10.0)	-	
BCVA(logMAR), n (%)	0.3< * ≤0.0	23 (76.7)	20 (66.7)	20 (100.0)	0.017 [3]
	1.0≤ * ≤0.3	7 (23.3)	10 (33.3)	0	

* BCVA score. [1] $F_{(2,76)}$ = 10.770; [2] $X^2_{(2)}$ = 2.979; [3] $X^2_{(2)}$ = 8.092. Data were expressed as mean and standard deviation where the analysis of variance was used for comparisons unless specified as number (percentage) using the Pearson χ^2 test or the Fisher–Freeman–Halton test as appropriate. A p value of less than 0.05 was considered significant. Abbreviations: BCVA, best corrected visual acuity; CSC, central serous chorioretinopathy; CT, choroidal thickness.

At the time of data collection, all patients were treatment naive. Different treatment modalities were applied after plasma samples were collected.

Data on the plasma levels of angiogenic factors in patients with acute and chronic CSC as well as controls are shown in Table 3.

Table 3. Plasma levels of angiogenic factors in patients with acute and chronic central serous chorioretinopathy as well as controls.

Angiogenic Factor, pg/mL	Acute CSC (n = 30)	Chronic CSC (n = 30)	Controls (n = 20)	p Value
PEDF	94.99 (47.91–200.92)	82.89 (45.73–155.99)	74.12 (54.45–159.35)	0.80 [1]
FGF-basic	48.97 (2.74)	48.97 (4.71)	50.49 (3.11)	0.28 [2]
Endostatin	18,009.97 (4466.25)	18,241.17 (4524.54)	16,854.20 (3182.28)	0.49 [3]
FGF-acid	127.40 (7.92)	125.20 (8.11)	126.08 (8.20)	0.58 [4]
PDGF-AA	179.04 (87.66)	200.23 (143.25)	265.19 (97.72)	0.03 [5]
PlGF	3.40 (0.76)	3.44 (0.91)	3.99 (0.96)	0.045 [6]
VEGF-D	78.62 (5.88)	76.93 (9.66)	77.94 (6.99)	0.70 [7]
Trombospondin-2	4661.00 (4070.00–6002.00)	5478.00 (5420.00–6933.00)	5898.00 (4750.00–6857.00)	0.07 [8]
Angiopoietin-1	2894.00 (1722.00–3760.00)	2373.00 (1321.00–2943.00)	3982.00 (2411.00–5617.00)	0.01 [9]
VEGF	8.80 (6.00-14.40)	9.40 (6.60-13.10)	14.50 (8.60-23.00)	0.07 [10]

[1] $X^2_{(2)}$ = 0.447; [2] $F_{(2,77)}$ = 1.275; [3] $F_{(2,77)}$ = 0.707; [4] $F_{(2,76)}$ = 0.553; [5] $F_{(2,77)}$ = 3.558; [6] $F_{(2,77)}$ = 3.230; [7] $F_{(2,77)}$ = 0.359; [8] $X^2_{(2)}$ = 5.248; [9] $X^2_{(2)}$ = 9.656; [10] $X^2_{(2)}$ = 5.091. Data are shown as mean and standard deviation where the analysis of variance was used for comparisons or as median (interquartile range) using the Kruskal-Wallis test for comparison. A p value of less than 0.05 was considered significant. Abbreviations: CSC, central serous chorioretinopathy; FGF, fibroblast growth factor; PEDF, pigment epithelium–derived factor; PDGF, platelet-derived growth factor; PlGF, placental growth factor; VEGF, vascular endothelial growth factor.

Intergroup comparisons of the plasma levels of the 10 measured angiogenic factors revealed significant differences between the study groups for angiopoietin-1, PlGF, and PDGF-AA (Figure 1a–c). There were no differences in the levels of the remaining antiangiogenic factors among the three groups (p > 0.05).

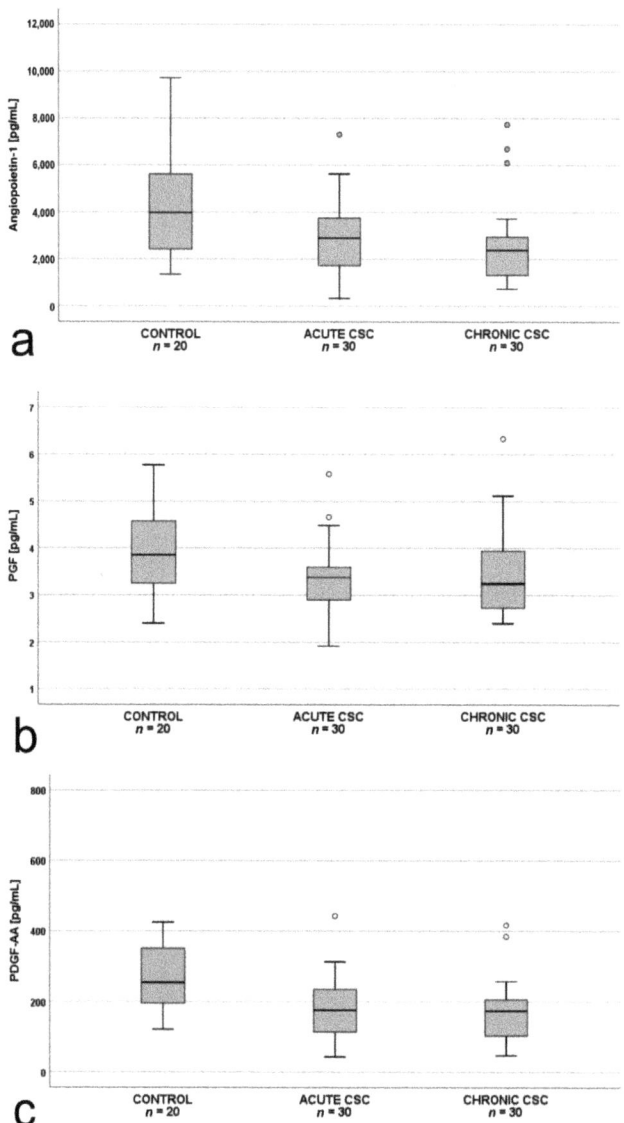

Figure 1. Box-and-whisker plot of: (**a**) plasma angiopoietin-1 ($p = 0.01$; $X^2(2) = 9.656$); (**b**) placental growth factor (PlGF; $p = 0.045$; $F(2.77) = 3.230$); and (**c**) plasma pigment epithelium–derived factor (PDGF-AA; $p = 0.03$; $F(2.77) = 3.558$) levels in patients with acute central serous chorioretinopathy, patients with chronic central serous chorioretinopathy and controls. The line inside the box represents the median; the lower and upper sides of the box represent the lower and upper quartiles, respectively. Whiskers represent cases distant up to 1.5 of interquartile range (IQR) from the respective quartile; circles, cases distant from 1.5 to 3 IQRs. p values were estimated using the analysis of variance for normally distributed variables and the Kruskal–Wallis test otherwise.

Subsequent pairwise comparisons showed that in patients with acute CSC ($n = 30$), plasma PDGF-AA levels were significantly lower than in the controls ($n = 20$) (Figure 2), whereas in patients with chronic CSC ($n = 30$), angiopoietin-1 levels were significantly lower than in the controls ($n = 20$) (Figure 3).

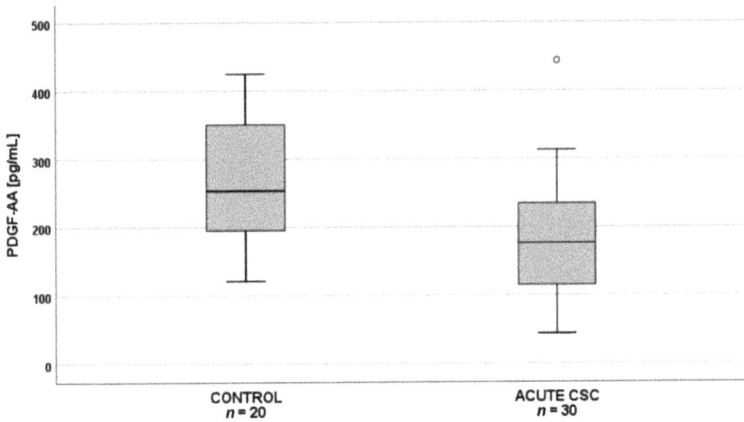

Figure 2. Box-and-whisker plot of plasma pigment epithelium–derived factor (PDGF-AA) levels in patients with acute central serous chorioretinopathy and controls ($p = 0.002$; $t(48) = 3.252$). The line inside the box represents the median; the lower and upper sides of the box represent the lower and upper quartiles, respectively. Whiskers represent cases distant up to 1.5 of interquartile range (IQR) from the respective quartile; circles, cases distant from 1.5 to 3 IQRs. p values were estimated using the analysis of variance post-hoc Bonferroni test.

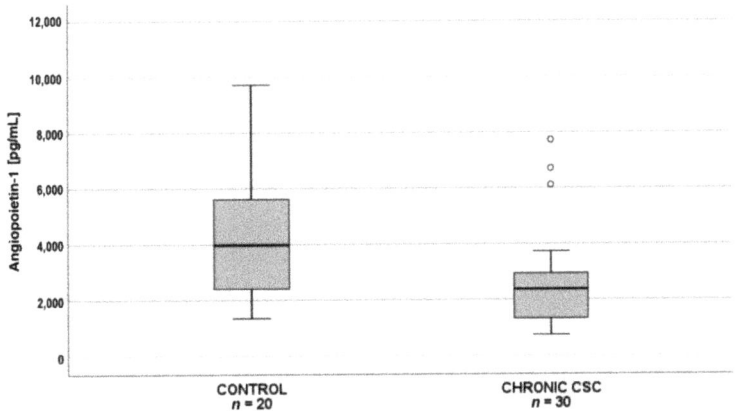

Figure 3. Box-and-whisker plot of plasma angiopoietin-1 levels in patients with chronic central serous chorioretinopathy and controls ($p = 0.007$; $X^2(2) = 9.656$; post hoc test statistics = 20.3). The line inside the box represents the median; the lower and upper sides of the box represent the lower and upper quartiles, respectively. Whiskers represent cases distant up to 1.5 of interquartile range (IQR) from the respective quartile; circles, cases distant from 1.5 to 3 IQRs. p values were estimated using the post-hoc pairwise comparison for the Kruskal–Wallis test with Bonferroni correction.

Additionally, we performed an analysis for the whole CSC group (patients with both chronic and acute form, $n = 60$) vs. controls ($n = 20$). Plasma VEGF, PDGF-AA, and PlGF levels in patients with acute or chronic CSC ($n = 60$) were significantly lower than in the controls (Figure 4a–c).

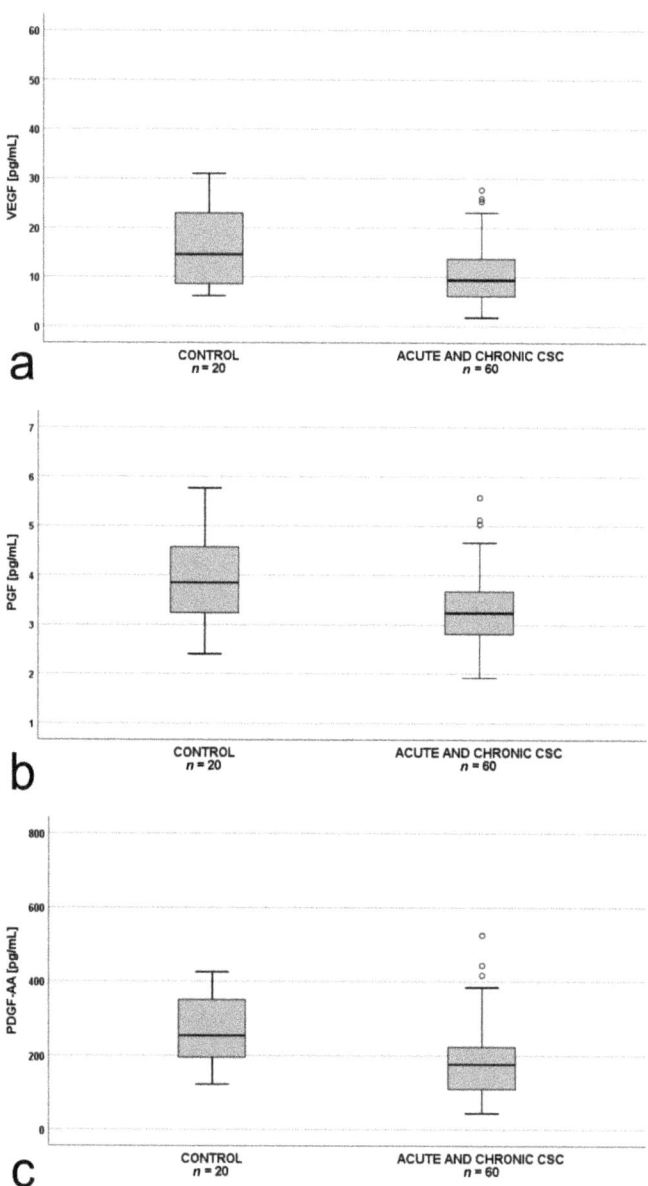

Figure 4. Box-and-whisker plot of: (**a**) plasma vascular endothelial growth factor (VEGF; $p = 0.024$); (**b**) plasma placental growth factor (PlGF; $p = 0.013$; $t(48) = -2.551$); (**c**) platelet-derived growth factor AA (PDGF-AA; $p = 0.012$; $t(48) = -2.577$) levels in all patients with central serous chorioretinopathy (acute and chronic) and controls. The line inside the box represents the median; the lower and upper sides of the box represent the lower and upper quartiles, respectively. Whiskers represent cases distant up to 1.5 of interquartile range (IQR) from the respective quartile; circles, cases distant from 1.5 to 3 IQRs. p values were estimated using the t-test for normally distributed variables and the Mann–Whitney test otherwise.

The analysis of the correlation between mean CT and VEGF for the whole CSC cohort ($n = 60$) revealed an inverse correlation, which was particularly prominent after exclusion of a single outlier in VEGF measurement (>50 pg/mL) (Figure 5a). Further analysis proved that this correlation was true for patients with chronic CSC (Figure 5b), but was not observed in the acute-CSC group ($rho = 0.07$, $p = 0.721$).

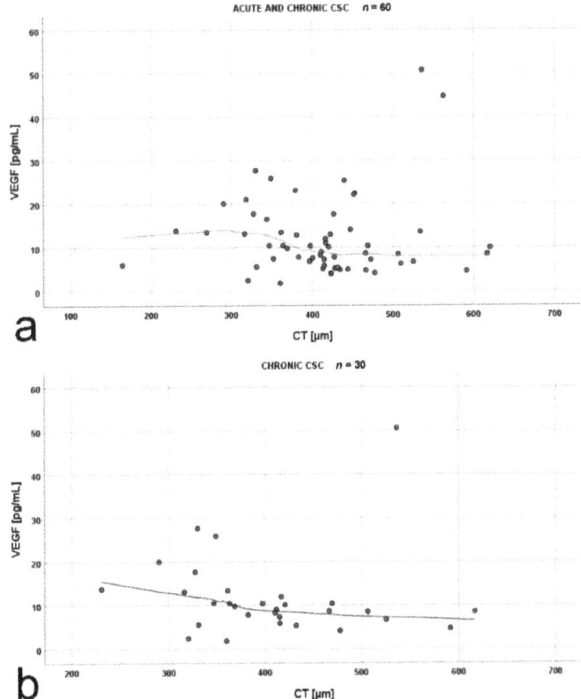

Figure 5. Scatterplots showing the correlations between: (**a**) mean choroidal thickness (CT) and vascular endothelial growth factor (VEGF) levels in patients with acute and chronic central serous chorioretinopathy ($rho = -0.27$, $p = 0.044$); (**b**) mean CT and VEGF levels in patients with chronic central serous chorioretinopathy ($rho = -0.48$, $p = 0.009$). The strength of the relationship between the variables was estimated using the Spearman rank correlation coefficient *rho*. The shape of the relationship was presented using the loess curve.

4. Discussion

Choroidal vasculature plays a crucial role in retinal homeostasis and preservation of good vision and vision-related Quality of Life [27]. Importantly, the key pathophysiologic mechanism in CSC is associated with the presence of abnormally thick choroid, hyperpermeable, and dilated choroidal vessels with or without RPE abnormalities overlying the pachyvessels [7]. Dysregulation in angiogenesis and arteriogenesis has been suggested as an underlying mechanism for the development of some chorioretinal diseases [3,19].

Angiogenesis is a highly controlled process involving the formation of new blood vessels from a preexisting vascular bed and depends on an intricate balance of both proangiogenic and antiangiogenic factors. On the other hand, arteriogenesis refers to anatomic transformation of preexisting arterioles, with an increase in the lumen area and wall thickness, due to a thick muscular layer and development of viscoelastic and vasomotor capacities [25]. The two processes differ in several aspects, with the most important being that angiogenesis depends on hypoxia and arteriogenesis on inflammation [25]. Based on these facts, it may be suspected that there is a relationship between the pathogenesis of pachychoroid diseases, especially CSC, and the levels of angiogenic factors in human blood.

To the best of our knowledge, this is the first study that assessed the plasma levels of angiogenic factors such as angiopoietin-1, endostatin, FGF-acidic, FGF-basic, PlGF, PDGF-AA, thrombospondin-2, VEGF, VEGF-D, and PEDF in patients with CSC in comparison with heathy individuals. We noted differences in the plasma levels of angiopoietin-1, PlGF, and PDGF-AA between patients with acute and chronic CSC as well as the controls. The levels of PDGF-AA were downregulated only in acute CSC, whereas those of angiopoietin-1 only in chronic CSC, compared with the controls.

It has been shown that angiopoietin-1 is essential for vessel stabilization and quiescence in adults [28]. In this context, Lee et al. [29] found that the interendothelial junctional protein reduced recruitment and infiltration of macrophages from the Bruch's membrane, thus preventing CNV formation and consecutive vascular leakage. Interestingly, a dysregulated interaction between the RPE and infiltrated macrophages results in upregulation of angiogenesis and leads to choroidal abnormalities in chronic CSC [30]. Terao et al. [30] reported that inflammation, accompanied by macrophage infiltration, into the choroid and retina may cause CSC progression from the acute to chronic form. Angiopoietin-1 is also known to support endothelial cell stabilization by activating the Tie-2 receptor and to decrease vascular leakage by increasing the level of the interendothelial cell junction proteins [29]. Previous studies revealed that angiopoietin-1 prevents the VEGF-A–mediated junction disruption [21]; however, a recent report indicated that it may directly stabilize vascular endothelial cadherin and zonula occludens-1 by regulating the RhoA-specific guanine nucleotide exchange factor Syx [31]. Noteworthy, administration of angiopoietin-1 into the vitreous body upregulates the expression of vascular endothelial cadherin and zonula occludens-1, the key factors of endothelial cell-to-cell junctions preserving vascular integrity [28,32]. We hypothesized that the deficiency of angiopoietin-1 demonstrated in our study may result in dissociation of endothelial tight junctions in the choriocapillaris and choroid, leading to chronic vascular dysfunction associated with the prolonged presence of the serous retinal detachment and/or fluid under the RPE in the course of chronic CSC.

Schubert et al. [33] postulated that structural and molecular changes in the choriocapillaris and choroid in CSC can alter the microenvironment of the RPE. This, in turn, can affect RPE barrier capabilities and its transport [33]. The endothelial cells of the choriocapillaris are fenestrated; therefore, they have higher permeability than the nonfenestrated retinal capillaries. This may suggest that even in physiological conditions, the RPE is regularly exposed to plasma filtrate [33]. In our study, the plasma concentrations of PlGF and PDGF-AA were downregulated in patients with CSC compared with the controls. Placental growth factor is a multifunctional cytokine affecting diverse cellular activities [34]. Its pleiotropic effects on junction stabilization, survival, proliferation, and metabolism as well activation effects on vascular cells (i.e., pericytes and smooth muscle cells, endothelial cells) were reported [34]. There is an increasing body of evidence showing that lowering or elevating PlGF expression may lead to various diseases [34]. Moreover, PlGF increases the expression of some angiogenic factors such as VEGF, PDGF-B, and FGF-2 [29], which stimulate angiogenesis through proliferation of endothelial cells and arteriogenesis through smooth muscles [35].

Platelet-derived growth factor stimulates both arteriogenesis and angiogenesis [25]. Tumor growth factor-β produced by different cells is a chemoattractant for monocytes. It also stimulates the expression of PDGF by these cells during arteriogenesis [35], which may be involved in the development of CNV in chronic CSC [36]. The deficiency of PDGF in acute CSC may explain the absence of CNV, but this hypothesis merits further research. Saito et al. [37] confirmed that PDGF-AA was crucial for retina regeneration within the first hours after injury; therefore, its deficiency may play a role in the acute form of CSC.

In our study, the VEGF was significantly downregulated in patients with CSC (both acute and chronic) compared with the controls. Only a few studies assessed angiogenic factors in plasma and aqueous humor (AH) of patients with CSC. Lim et al. [38] did not show any differences in plasma and AH levels of VEGF in CSC compared with the controls. However, the study was limited by a small group of patients, mostly with acute CSC, which precluded a definitive conclusion. Shin et al. [39] reported similar, but very low, AH levels of VEGF in patients with CSC and the controls, but PDGF levels were lower in CSC.

Downregulated plasma VEGF levels in CSC compared with the healthy individuals observed in our study may partially explain an unsatisfactory effect of intravitreal anti-VEGF treatment in patients with CSC [2,40]. Even though CSC is described as a vascular disorder (pachychoroid), the primary exudative component leading to a macular detachment is considered to be nonvasogenic, which means that it does not result directly from the proliferation of choroidal vessels [8,41]. This is an essential difference between CSC and other conditions presenting with serous macular detachment and CNV such as nAMD [8,41,42].

The fact that chronic CSC can be associated with the presence of CNV [16,17] does not contradict the results of our study, which revealed lower plasma VEGF levels in CSC patients compared with the controls. This is in line with the studies by Spaide et al. [36] and Sacconi et al. [43]. They hypothesized that CNV in CSC occurs as a result of proliferation of new vessels during arteriogenesis, which is characterized by dilation of the existing vascular channels and is independent of VEGF (unlike angiogenesis, which is highly VEGF dependent) [44]. On the other hand, VEGF alters the junctional integrity, downregulates the expression of occludin and zonula occludens-1 [45–48], which results in increased permeability and angiogenesis [15,49]. Downregulated VEGF levels observed in our study may suggest that the mechanism of vascular hyperpermeability in CSC is similar to that of CNV in VEGF independent CSC and may result from altered flow in dilated choroidal vessels (pachyvessels) [7]. The increased flow leads to endothelial cell proliferation, with luminar expansion and release of platelet endothelial cell adhesion molecule-1, monocyte chemoattractant protein-1, intracellular adhesion molecule-1, and vascular cell adhesion molecule-1 [50]. As a result, increased endothelial permeability, as indicated by the leakage of plasma proteins, erythrocytes, and platelets into the vascular wall and the adherence of monocytes to the endothelium, was observed, along with the recruitment of circulating monocytes and resident macrophages [51]. This, in turn, promotes arteriogenesis by the ability of monocytes and macrophages to secrete metalloproteinases, chemokines, and growth factors [25,52].

We hypothesized that the impaired function of RPE cells in CSC, a major source of ocular proangiogenic proteins, may result in decreased intraocular levels of VEGF, but it does not fully explain the downregulation of the other analyzed proangiogenic factors in the eyes, especially in plasma. This issue merits further investigation.

In the current study, we did not find differences in the levels of antiangiogenic proteins, trombospondin-2, and endostatin between patients with CSC and the controls. It is well known that antihypertensive drugs affect angiogenesis [53,54]. However, in our study, we did not observe any differences in the levels of proangiogenic and antiangiogenic factors between patients using at least one antihypertensive drug and those not receiving any medication. This finding requires further research.

In our study, an inverse correlation between mean CT and VEGF was observed in chronic CSC. It was shown that a decrease in VEGF levels in intraocular fluids as a result of intravitreal anti-VEGF therapy leads to a decrease in CT in patients with diabetic retinopathy [55]. Furthermore, some studies reported a decrease in CT in patients with acute CSC after anti-VEGF treatment [56]. These data suggest that certain levels of VEGF are necessary to maintain choroidal stability and function, which is also in line with our results. Nevertheless, this is an interesting phenomenon that definitely deserves a more substantial discussion and more thorough research.

Our study was limited by the fact that it was performed at a single time point and only plasma, and not AH, samples were investigated. Moreover, there were possible confounding factors affecting the levels of angiogenic factors such as concomitant antihypertensive treatment. Finally, during blood sample collection, we did not record the stage of the menstruation cycle in women at reproductive age, while menstruation cycle is known to affect angiogenic markers. Although the lack of AH assessment may be an important limitation, the significant differences in the plasma levels of angiogenic factors are an interesting finding, indicating that CSC might be a systemic disease.

5. Conclusions

Downregulated angiopoietin-1, VEGF, PDGF-AA, and PlGF levels observed in our study may highlight the previously unknown role of the imbalanced levels of proangiogenic and antiangiogenic factors, which affect choroidal hyperpermeability and exert profound changes in venular structure and function, thus possibly contributing to the pathogenesis of CSC. Lower plasma levels of VEGF in patients with CSC may support the hypothesis that CNV occurs in these patients as a result of arteriogenesis, which is less VEGF-dependent than angiogenesis. Moreover, our findings may support the search for new therapeutic strategies in CSC. Nevertheless, the underlying mechanisms that contribute to this condition remain largely unknown and require further studies.

Author Contributions: Conceptualization, I.K.-B. and M.S.; Methodology, I.K.-B. and M.S.; Software, M.G.; Validation, I.K.-B. and B.R.-D.; Formal analysis, I.K.-B. and W.P.-M.; Investigation, I.K.-B., W.P.-M., M.C. and A.K.-T.; Resources, I.K.-B., W.P.-M. and M.D.-K.; Data curation, I.K.-B.; Writing—original draft preparation, I.K.-B., W.P.-M. and M.D.-K.; Writing—review and editing, M.G. and M.S.; Visualization, I.K.-B., W.P.-M. and M.C.; Supervision, B.R.-D. and M.S.; Project administration, W.P.-M.; Funding acquisition, I.K.-B. All authors have read and agreed to the published version of the manuscript.

Funding: This research was funded by Jagiellonian University Medical College, Krakow, Poland, grant no. K/ZDS/006283; to I.K.-B.). The APC was funded by the authors.

Institutional Review Board Statement: The study was conducted according to the guidelines of the Declaration of Helsinki and approved by the Ethics Committee of Jagiellonian University in Krakow, Poland (protocol codes 122.6120.266.2016; 27 October 2016).

Informed Consent Statement: Informed consent was obtained from all subjects involved in the study.

Data Availability Statement: Not applicable.

Acknowledgments: Not applicable.

Conflicts of Interest: The authors declare no conflict of interest.

References

1. Van Rijssen, T.J.; van Dijk, E.H.C.; Yzer, S.; Ohno-Matsui, K.; Keunen, J.E.E.; Schlingemann, R.O.; Sivaprasad, S.; Querques, G.; Downes, S.M.; Fauser, S.; et al. Central serous chorioretinopathy: Towards an evidence-based treatment guideline. *Prog. Retin. Eye Res.* **2019**, 100770. [CrossRef]
2. Chung, Y.-R.; Seo, E.J.; Lew, H.M.; Lee, K.H. Lack of positive effect of intravitreal bevacizumab in central serous chorioretinopathy: Meta-analysis and review. *Eye Lond. Engl.* **2013**, *27*, 1339–1346. [CrossRef]
3. Sartini, F.; Figus, M.; Nardi, M.; Casini, G.; Posarelli, C. Non-resolving, recurrent and chronic central serous chorioretinopathy: Available treatment options. *Eye Lond. Engl.* **2019**, *33*, 1035–1043. [CrossRef]
4. Vilela, M.; Mengue, C. Central Serous Chorioretinopathy Classification. *Pharmaceuticals* **2020**, *14*, 26. [CrossRef]
5. Daruich, A.; Matet, A.; Dirani, A.; Bousquet, E.; Zhao, M.; Farman, N.; Jaisser, F.; Behar-Cohen, F. Central serous chorioretinopathy: Recent findings and new physiopathology hypothesis. *Prog. Retin. Eye Res.* **2015**, *48*, 82–118. [CrossRef] [PubMed]
6. Gawęcki, M.; Jaszczuk-Maciejewska, A.; Jurska-Jaśko, A.; Kneba, M.; Grzybowski, A. Impairment of visual acuity and retinal morphology following resolved chronic central serous chorioretinopathy. *BMC Ophthalmol.* **2019**, *19*, 160. [CrossRef] [PubMed]
7. Cheung, C.M.G.; Lee, W.K.; Koizumi, H.; Dansingani, K.; Lai, T.Y.Y.; Freund, K.B. Pachychoroid disease. *Eye Lond. Engl.* **2019**, *33*, 14–33. [CrossRef] [PubMed]
8. Sakurada, Y.; Leong, B.C.S.; Parikh, R.; Fragiotta, S.; Freund, K.B. Association between choroidal caverns and choroidal vascular hyperpermeability in eyes with pachychoroid diseases. *Retina Phila. Pa* **2018**, *38*, 1977–1983. [CrossRef]
9. Karska-Basta, I.; Pociej-Marciak, W.; Chrzaszcz, M.; Wilanska, J.; Jager, M.J.; Markiewicz, A.; Romanowska-Dixon, B.; Sanak, M.; Kubicka-Trzaska, A. Differences in anti-endothelial and anti-retinal antibody titers: Implications for the pathohysiology of acute and chronic central serous chorioretinopathy. *J. Physiol. Pharmacol. Off. J. Pol. Physiol. Soc.* **2020**, *71*. [CrossRef]

10. Cheung, C.M.G.; Lai, T.Y.Y.; Ruamviboonsuk, P.; Chen, S.-J.; Chen, Y.; Freund, K.B.; Gomi, F.; Koh, A.H.; Lee, W.-K.; Wong, T.Y. Polypoidal Choroidal Vasculopathy: Definition, Pathogenesis, Diagnosis, and Management. *Ophthalmology* **2018**, *125*, 708–724. [CrossRef]
11. Kato, Y.; Oguchi, Y.; Omori, T.; Shintake, H.; Tomita, R.; Kasai, A.; Ogasawara, M.; Sugano, Y.; Itagaki, K.; Ojima, A.; et al. Complement Activation Products and Cytokines in Pachychoroid Neovasculopathy and Neovascular Age-Related Macular Degeneration. *Invest. Ophthalmol. Vis. Sci.* **2020**, *61*, 39. [CrossRef]
12. Hosoda, Y.; Yoshikawa, M.; Miyake, M.; Tabara, Y.; Ahn, J.; Woo, S.J.; Honda, S.; Sakurada, Y.; Shiragami, C.; Nakanishi, H.; et al. CFH and VIPR2 as susceptibility loci in choroidal thickness and pachychoroid disease central serous chorioretinopathy. *Proc. Natl. Acad. Sci. USA* **2018**, *115*, 6261–6266. [CrossRef]
13. Sartini, F.; Figus, M.; Casini, G.; Nardi, M.; Posarelli, C. Pachychoroid neovasculopathy: A type-1 choroidal neovascularization belonging to the pachychoroid spectrum-pathogenesis, imaging and available treatment options. *Int. Ophthalmol.* **2020**, *40*, 3577–3589. [CrossRef]
14. Sartini, F.; Menchini, M.; Posarelli, C.; Casini, G.; Figus, M. Bullous Central Serous Chorioretinopathy: A Rare and Atypical Form of Central Serous Chorioretinopathy. A Systematic Review. *Pharmaceuticals* **2020**, *13*, 221. [CrossRef] [PubMed]
15. Karska-Basta, I.; Pociej-Marciak, W.; Chrząszcz, M.; Kubicka-Trząska, A.; Romanowska-Dixon, B.; Sanak, M. Altered plasma cytokine levels in acute and chronic central serous chorioretinopathy. *Acta Ophthalmol.* **2020**. [CrossRef] [PubMed]
16. Shiragami, C.; Takasago, Y.; Osaka, R.; Kobayashi, M.; Ono, A.; Yamashita, A.; Hirooka, K. Clinical Features of Central Serous Chorioretinopathy With Type 1 Choroidal Neovascularization. *Am. J. Ophthalmol.* **2018**, *193*, 80–86. [CrossRef]
17. Mrejen, S.; Balaratnasingam, C.; Kaden, T.R.; Bottini, A.; Dansingani, K.; Bhavsar, K.V.; Yannuzzi, N.A.; Patel, S.; Chen, K.C.; Yu, S.; et al. Long-term Visual Outcomes and Causes of Vision Loss in Chronic Central Serous Chorioretinopathy. *Ophthalmology* **2019**, *126*, 576–588. [CrossRef]
18. Van Bergen, T.; Etienne, I.; Cunningham, F.; Moons, L.; Schlingemann, R.O.; Feyen, J.H.M.; Stitt, A.W. The role of placental growth factor (PlGF) and its receptor system in retinal vascular diseases. *Prog. Retin. Eye Res.* **2019**, *69*, 116–136. [CrossRef]
19. Muether, P.S.; Neuhann, I.; Buhl, C.; Hermann, M.M.; Kirchhof, B.; Fauser, S. Intraocular growth factors and cytokines in patients with dry and neovascular age-related macular degeneration. *Retina Phila. Pa* **2013**, *33*, 1809–1814. [CrossRef] [PubMed]
20. Siedlecki, J.; Wertheimer, C.; Wolf, A.; Liegl, R.; Priglinger, C.; Priglinger, S.; Eibl-Lindner, K. Combined VEGF and PDGF inhibition for neovascular AMD: Anti-angiogenic properties of axitinib on human endothelial cells and pericytes in vitro. *Graefes Arch. Clin. Exp. Ophthalmol. Albrecht Von Graefes Arch. Klin. Exp. Ophthalmol.* **2017**, *255*, 963–972. [CrossRef] [PubMed]
21. Gavard, J.; Patel, V.; Gutkind, J.S. Angiopoietin-1 prevents VEGF-induced endothelial permeability by sequestering Src through mDia. *Dev. Cell* **2008**, *14*, 25–36. [CrossRef]
22. Nagy, J.A.; Benjamin, L.; Zeng, H.; Dvorak, A.M.; Dvorak, H.F. Vascular permeability, vascular hyperpermeability and angiogenesis. *Angiogenesis* **2008**, *11*, 109–119. [CrossRef]
23. Farnoodian, M.; Wang, S.; Dietz, J.; Nickells, R.W.; Sorenson, C.M.; Sheibani, N. Negative regulators of angiogenesis: Important targets for treatment of exudative AMD. *Clin. Sci. Lond. Engl. 1979* **2017**, *131*, 1763–1780. [CrossRef] [PubMed]
24. Kuwano, M.; Fukushi, J.; Okamoto, M.; Nishie, A.; Goto, H.; Ishibashi, T.; Ono, M. Angiogenesis factors. *Intern. Med. Tokyo Jpn.* **2001**, *40*, 565–572. [CrossRef] [PubMed]
25. Rizzi, A.; Benagiano, V.; Ribatti, D. Angiogenesis versus arteriogenesis. *Rom. J. Morphol. Embryol. Rev. Roum. Morphol. Embryol.* **2017**, *58*, 15–19.
26. Branchini, L.A.; Adhi, M.; Regatieri, C.V.; Nandakumar, N.; Liu, J.J.; Laver, N.; Fujimoto, J.G.; Duker, J.S. Analysis of choroidal morphologic features and vasculature in healthy eyes using spectral-domain optical coherence tomography. *Ophthalmology* **2013**, *120*, 1901–1908. [CrossRef] [PubMed]
27. Karska-Basta, I.; Pociej-Marciak, W.; Chrząszcz, M.; Żuber-Łaskawiec, K.; Sanak, M.; Romanowska-Dixon, B. Quality of life of patients with central serous chorioretinopathy—A major cause of vision threat among middle-aged individuals. *Arch. Med. Sci.* **2020**, *16*. [CrossRef]
28. El-Asrar, M.A.; Elbarbary, N.S.; Ismail, E.A.R.; Bakr, A.A. Circulating angiopoietin-2 levels in children and adolescents with type 1 diabetes mellitus: Relation to carotid and aortic intima-media thickness. *Angiogenesis* **2016**, *19*, 421–431. [CrossRef] [PubMed]
29. Lee, J.; Park, D.-Y.; Park, D.Y.; Park, I.; Chang, W.; Nakaoka, Y.; Komuro, I.; Yoo, O.-J.; Koh, G.Y. Angiopoietin-1 suppresses choroidal neovascularization and vascular leakage. *Invest. Ophthalmol. Vis. Sci.* **2014**, *55*, 2191–2199. [CrossRef]
30. Terao, N.; Koizumi, H.; Kojima, K.; Yamagishi, T.; Nagata, K.; Kitazawa, K.; Yamamoto, Y.; Yoshii, K.; Hiraga, A.; Toda, M.; et al. Association of Upregulated Angiogenic Cytokines With Choroidal Abnormalities in Chronic Central Serous Chorioretinopathy. *Invest. Ophthalmol. Vis. Sci.* **2018**, *59*, 5924–5931. [CrossRef]
31. Ngok, S.P.; Geyer, R.; Liu, M.; Kourtidis, A.; Agrawal, S.; Wu, C.; Seerapu, H.R.; Lewis-Tuffin, L.J.; Moodie, K.L.; Huveldt, D.; et al. VEGF and Angiopoietin-1 exert opposing effects on cell junctions by regulating the Rho GEF Syx. *J. Cell Biol.* **2012**, *199*, 1103–1115. [CrossRef]
32. Peters, S.; Cree, I.A.; Alexander, R.; Turowski, P.; Ockrim, Z.; Patel, J.; Boyd, S.R.; Joussen, A.M.; Ziemssen, F.; Hykin, P.G.; et al. Angiopoietin modulation of vascular endothelial growth factor: Effects on retinal endothelial cell permeability. *Cytokine* **2007**, *40*, 144–150. [CrossRef]

33. Schubert, C.; Pryds, A.; Zeng, S.; Xie, Y.; Freund, K.B.; Spaide, R.F.; Merriam, J.C.; Barbazetto, I.; Slakter, J.S.; Chang, S.; et al. Cadherin 5 is regulated by corticosteroids and associated with central serous chorioretinopathy. *Hum. Mutat.* **2014**, *35*, 859–867. [CrossRef]
34. Dewerchin, M.; Carmeliet, P. PlGF: A multitasking cytokine with disease-restricted activity. *Cold Spring Harb. Perspect. Med.* **2012**, *2*. [CrossRef]
35. van Royen, N.; Piek, J.J.; Buschmann, I.; Hoefer, I.; Voskuil, M.; Schaper, W. Stimulation of arteriogenesis; a new concept for the treatment of arterial occlusive disease. *Cardiovasc. Res.* **2001**, *49*, 543–553. [CrossRef]
36. Spaide, R.F. Optical Coherence Tomography Angiography Signs of Vascular Abnormalization With Antiangiogenic Therapy for Choroidal Neovascularization. *Am. J. Ophthalmol.* **2015**, *160*, 6–16. [CrossRef]
37. Saito, M.; Saito, W.; Hirooka, K.; Hashimoto, Y.; Mori, S.; Noda, K.; Ishida, S. Pulse Waveform Changes in Macular Choroidal Hemodynamics With Regression of Acute Central Serous Chorioretinopathy. *Invest. Ophthalmol. Vis. Sci.* **2015**, *56*, 6515–6522. [CrossRef]
38. Lim, J.W.; Kim, M.U.; Shin, M.-C. Aqueous humor and plasma levels of vascular endothelial growth factor and interleukin-8 in patients with central serous chorioretinopathy. *Retina Phila. Pa* **2010**, *30*, 1465–1471. [CrossRef]
39. Shin, M.C.; Lim, J.W. Concentration of cytokines in the aqueous humor of patients with central serous chorioretinopathy. *Retina Phila. Pa* **2011**, *31*, 1937–1943. [CrossRef]
40. Ji, S.; Wei, Y.; Chen, J.; Tang, S. Clinical efficacy of anti-VEGF medications for central serous chorioretinopathy: A meta-analysis. *Int. J. Clin. Pharm.* **2017**, *39*, 514–521. [CrossRef]
41. Spaide, R.F.; Koizumi, H.; Pozzoni, M.C.; Pozonni, M.C. Enhanced depth imaging spectral-domain optical coherence tomography. *Am. J. Ophthalmol.* **2008**, *146*, 496–500. [CrossRef]
42. Żuber-Łaskawiec, K.; Kubicka-Trząska, A.; Karska-Basta, I.; Pociej-Marciak, W.; Romanowska-Dixon, B. Non-Responsiveness and Tachyphylaxis to Anti-Vascular Endothelial Growth Factor Treatment in Naive Patients with Exudative Age-Related Macular Degeneration. Available online: https://pubmed.ncbi.nlm.nih.gov/32009630/ (accessed on 2 December 2020).
43. Sacconi, R.; Tomasso, L.; Corbelli, E.; Carnevali, A.; Querques, L.; Casati, S.; Bandello, F.; Querques, G. Early response to the treatment of choroidal neovascularization complicating central serous chorioretinopathy: A OCT-angiography study. *Eye Lond. Engl.* **2019**, *33*, 1809–1817. [CrossRef] [PubMed]
44. Schierling, W.; Troidl, K.; Troidl, C.; Schmitz-Rixen, T.; Schaper, W.; Eitenmüller, I.K. The role of angiogenic growth factors in arteriogenesis. *J. Vasc. Res.* **2009**, *46*, 365–374. [CrossRef] [PubMed]
45. Behzadian, M.A.; Windsor, L.J.; Ghaly, N.; Liou, G.; Tsai, N.-T.; Caldwell, R.B. VEGF-induced paracellular permeability in cultured endothelial cells involves urokinase and its receptor. *FASEB J. Off. Publ. Fed. Am. Soc. Exp. Biol.* **2003**, *17*, 752–754. [CrossRef] [PubMed]
46. Liu, X.; Dreffs, A.; Díaz-Coránguez, M.; Runkle, E.A.; Gardner, T.W.; Chiodo, V.A.; Hauswirth, W.W.; Antonetti, D.A. Occludin S490 Phosphorylation Regulates Vascular Endothelial Growth Factor-Induced Retinal Neovascularization. *Am. J. Pathol.* **2016**, *186*, 2486–2499. [CrossRef] [PubMed]
47. Murakami, T.; Frey, T.; Lin, C.; Antonetti, D.A. Protein kinase cβ phosphorylates occludin regulating tight junction trafficking in vascular endothelial growth factor-induced permeability in vivo. *Diabetes* **2012**, *61*, 1573–1583. [CrossRef] [PubMed]
48. Yun, J.-H.; Park, S.W.; Kim, K.-J.; Bae, J.-S.; Lee, E.H.; Paek, S.H.; Kim, S.U.; Ye, S.; Kim, J.-H.; Cho, C.-H. Endothelial STAT3 Activation Increases Vascular Leakage Through Downregulating Tight Junction Proteins: Implications for Diabetic Retinopathy. *J. Cell. Physiol.* **2017**, *232*, 1123–1134. [CrossRef]
49. Mesquida, M.; Leszczynska, A.; Llorenç, V.; Adán, A. Interleukin-6 blockade in ocular inflammatory diseases. *Clin. Exp. Immunol.* **2014**, *176*, 301–309. [CrossRef]
50. Chen, Z.; Rubin, J.; Tzima, E. Role of PECAM-1 in arteriogenesis and specification of preexisting collaterals. *Circ. Res.* **2010**, *107*, 1355–1363. [CrossRef]
51. Takeda, Y.; Costa, S.; Delamarre, E.; Roncal, C.; Leite de Oliveira, R.; Squadrito, M.L.; Finisguerra, V.; Deschoemaeker, S.; Bruyère, F.; Wenes, M.; et al. Macrophage skewing by Phd2 haplodeficiency prevents ischaemia by inducing arteriogenesis. *Nature* **2011**, *479*, 122–126. [CrossRef]
52. Galis, Z.S.; Sukhova, G.K.; Libby, P. Microscopic localization of active proteases by in situ zymography: Detection of matrix metalloproteinase activity in vascular tissue. *FASEB J. Off. Publ. Fed. Am. Soc. Exp. Biol.* **1995**, *9*, 974–980. [CrossRef]
53. Humar, R.; Zimmerli, L.; Battegay, E. Angiogenesis and hypertension: An update. *J. Hum. Hypertens.* **2009**, *23*, 773–782. [CrossRef]
54. Pociej-Marciak, W.; Karska-Basta, I.; Kuźniewski, M.; Kubicka-Trząska, A.; Romanowska-Dixon, B. Sudden visual deterioration as a first symptom of chronic kidney failure. *Case Rep Ophtalmol.* **2015**, *28*, 394–400. [CrossRef]
55. Kniggendorf, V.F.; Novais, E.A.; Kniggendorf, S.L.; Xavier, C.; Cole, E.D.; Regatieri, C.V. Effect of intravitreal anti-VEGF on choroidal thickness in patients with diabetic macular edema using spectral domain OCT. *Arq. Bras. Oftalmol.* **2016**, *79*, 155–158. [CrossRef]
56. Kim, D.Y.; Joe, S.G.; Yang, H.S.; Lee, J.Y.; Kim, J.-G.; Yoon, Y.H. Subfoveal choroidal thickness changes in treated idiopathic central serous chorioretinopathy and their association with recurrence. *Retina Phila. Pa* **2015**, *35*, 1867–1874. [CrossRef]

Idiopathic Peripheral Retinal Telangiectasia in Adults: A Case Series and Literature Review

Maciej Gawęcki

Dobry Wzrok Ophthalmological Clinic, 80-822 Gdansk, Poland; maciej@gawecki.com; Tel.: +48-501-788-654

Abstract: Idiopathic peripheral retinal telangiectasia (IPT), often termed as Coats disease, can present in a milder form with the onset in adulthood. The goal of this case series study and literature review was to describe and classify different presenting forms and treatment of this entity and to review contemporary methods of its management. Six cases of adult onset IPT were described with the following phenotypes based on fundus ophthalmoscopy, fluorescein angiography, and optical coherence tomography findings: IPT without exudates or foveal involvement, IPT with peripheral exudates without foveal involvement, IPT with peripheral exudates and cystoid macular edema, and IPT with peripheral and macular hard exudates. Treatments applied in this series included observation, laser photocoagulation, and anti-vascular endothelial growth factor (VEGF) treatment with variable outcomes depending upon the extent of IPT, the aggressiveness of laser treatment, and the stringency of follow-up. The accompanying literature review suggests that ablative therapies, especially laser photocoagulation, remain the most effective treatment option in adult-onset IPT, with anti-VEGF therapy serving as an adjuvant procedure. Close follow-up is necessary to achieve and maintain reasonable good visual and morphological results.

Keywords: Coats disease; peripheral retinal telangiectasia; laser photocoagulation; anti-VEGF treatment

1. Introduction

Idiopathic peripheral retinal telangiectasia (IPT), usually referred to as Coats disease, has been well-described in the medical literature since its discovery in 1908 [1]. Coats disease is an idiopathic condition characterized by telangiectatic and aneurysmal retinal vessels with intraretinal and subretinal exudation and fluid without appreciable retinal or vitreal traction, frequently associated with retinal detachment [2]. The pathogenesis and progression of that disease depends on the impairment of retinal vasculature. Alterations of endothelium of retinal vessels lead to breaking of blood-retinal barrier and presence of abnormal pericytes, causing formation of telangiectasias and closure of some vessels [3,4]. Exudation of lipids from the damaged vessels follows and is responsible for retinal detachment and cyst formation as well as retinal ischemia due to vessel closure [5]. The process is described as similar to pathogenesis of diabetic retinopathy, but definitely more severe and rapid [6].

Coats disease commonly presents unilaterally with strong male predominance. It has reportedly occurred in patients ranging from 4 months to 70 years of age, with the peak incidence in the first decade of life [5]. Its severe form (referred to as Coats disease) and milder form (sometimes termed Leber miliary aneurysms) that commonly present in adults, were initially described as separate entities [7]. Now, they are considered to be variable expressions of the same disease This explains its adult onset, as milder forms often stay asymptomatic for a long period of time [8,9]. Less severe forms of Coats disease fall into category 1, 2A and 2 B of the Shields classification commonly used to describe the stages of this disease [10]. Nevertheless, the perception of many ophthalmologists is that Coats disease is attributed to young children, only, and limited peripheral forms of this clinical entity are still frequently labeled differently, which causes inconsistencies in classification of the disease. Moreover, different systems of classification of retinal telangiectasia sometimes mix peripheral and central variants of the entity [11,12]. Terminology used to describe retinal telangiectasias together with their characteristics is provided in Table 1.

Table 1. Terminology used to describe idiopathic retinal telangiectasias.

Term	Characteristics
Coats disease	Idiopathic, nonhereditary aneurysmal retinal telangiectasia associated with intraretinal exudation and frequent exudative retinal detachment, occurring in patients aged a few months to seven decades with the peak in the first decade of life [2]
Leber miliary aneurysms	A milder variant of Coats disease, usually occurring in young adults and located at the retinal periphery [7–9]
Idiopathic retinal telangiectasia	A descriptive name for a Coats disease
MACTEL type 1	Macular telangiectasia type 1—aneurysmal type of macular telangiectasia, considered a central variant of Coats disease [13]
MACTEL type 2	Macular telangiectasia type 2—non-aneurysmal perifoveal capillary telangiectasia, associated with atrophy of neurosensory retina, presenting in the non-proliferative or proliferative form [13,14]

The diagnosis of IPT also can be challenging. Peripheral retinal telangiectasias accompany some rare systemic conditions, so before diagnosing the idiopathic form, it is important to rule out the primary underlying condition. Moreover, IPT is often asymptomatic and, as such, frequently missed, thus obscuring the real prevalence of the disease. On the other hand, if IPT results in macular edema and the far periphery of the retina is not examined, the condition might not be recognized as being secondary to the lesion located outside the posterior pole, leading to an erroneous therapeutic approach and sometimes lack of medical improvement.

Finally, there are numerous approaches to treatment for the different phenotypes of IPT, which have evolved in concert with progress in ophthalmology and the advent of new therapeutic methods.

The goal of this case series report was to present the different forms of presentation of IPT seen in an adult patient population as well as the observed responses to variable treatment modalities. Various diagnostic and therapeutic scenarios experienced by the author are placed in the perspective of available research from other clinicians.

2. Materials and Methods

A retrospective search of Dobry Wzrok clinic medical records was conducted to identify adult patients with peripheral telangiectasia confirmed by the results of fluorescein angiography (FA). Cases of aneurysmal macular telangiectasia (MACTEL type 1) as described in the classification of MACTEL proposed by Yanuzzi in 2006 were excluded from this study because they involved a centralized lesion location [13]. Additionally, a literature search was performed in the PubMed database for the phrase "peripheral retinal telangiectasias" and the combination of words "Coats disease" and "adult onset."

3. Results

The Dobry Wzrok clinic records contained six cases of idiopathic peripheral retinal telangiectasia in adults aged 21 to 60 years, including five men and one woman. In all cases, lesions were limited to one eye only and the other eye remained without compromise. Patient characteristics are presented in Table 2.

Table 2. Characteristics of patients with peripheral telangiectasias in this case series.

Case No/Gender	Proposed Category	Age (Years)	Eye, BCVA, Presentation of the Macula	Treatment	Follow-Up	Final BCVA and Disease State
1. M	1	20	RE, 20/20; no exudates, macular area normal	Observation	12 months	20/20; no progression
2. F	2	60	LE, 20/25; peripheral hard exudates, macular area normal	LPC in the periphery	12 months	20/25; no progression
3. M	3	20	LE, 20/60; peripheral hard exudates, CME without exudates	LPC in the periphery, intravitreal anti-VEGF	12 months	20/30; remission of CME
4. M	3	44	RE, 20/25; demarcated peripheral hard exudates, mild CME without exudates	LPC in the periphery, intravitreal anti-VEGF	20 months	20/80; progression of CME despite treatment
5. M	3	55	RE, 20/100; asteroid hyalosis, localized hard exudates outside the fovea, CME without exudates; risk of macular hole formation	LPC in the periphery	6 months	20/100; no improvement, intravitreal anti-VEGF scheduled, possible surgical treatment
6. M	4	21	LE, 6/200; peripheral and central hard exudates, CME	LPC in the periphery and GRID in the macula	12 months	20/20; remission of ME

M—male, F—female, RE—right eye, LE—left eye, BCVA—best-corrected visual acuity; CME—cystoid macular edema; LPC—laser photocoagulation; VEGF—vascular endothelial growth factor.

Study participants were divided into four categories depending on their presentation as follows:

- Category 1: IPT without peripheral exudates and without macular involvement (patient 1)
- Category 2: IPT with peripheral exudates and without macular involvement (patient 2)
- Category 3: IPT with peripheral exudates and cystoid macular edema without exudates (patients 3,4,5)
- Category 4: IPT with peripheral exudates and macular hard exudates and edema (patient 6)

3.1. Categories 1 and 2

Patients 1 and 2 were two cases of asymptomatic IPT found in our records search. In both cases, the length of follow-up was about 12 months. Both cases were asymptomatic—the lesions were found during routine ophthalmological examinations. Fundus examination and FA in both cases revealed IPT limited to a relatively small area of the peripheral retina. In one case, some amount of flat, hard exudates was observed at the border of the lesion, but macular edema was not present (patient 2) (Figure 1). In that case, laser photocoagulation (LPC) was applied to the IPT area (Figure 2). The other case was followed without any treatment; during the follow-up period, no telangiectasia progression was observed.

3.2. Category 3

Category 3 consisted of three cases of IPT that presented with mild to moderate macular cystoid edema without hard exudates (patients 3–5). All of these patients were symptomatic and complained of vision impairment in one eye. In all cases, the duration of symptoms was relatively short, according to the patients, at between one and three months. The diagnosis of IPT was confirmed by FA and macular edema was evaluated and monitored with spectral-domain optical coherence tomography (SD-OCT). Two cases (patients 3, 4) were treated with LPC of peripheral lesions combined with intravitreal bevacizumab or aflibercept injections. One patient (patient 5) underwent LPC and was scheduled for anti-vascular endothelial growth factor (VEGF) treatment. In one case (patient 3), complete remission of CME was noted after 12 months of follow-up; his BCVA remained stable at the level of 20/30 and did not improve further. FA photographs and SD-OCT scans before and after treatment are presented in Figures 3 and 4.

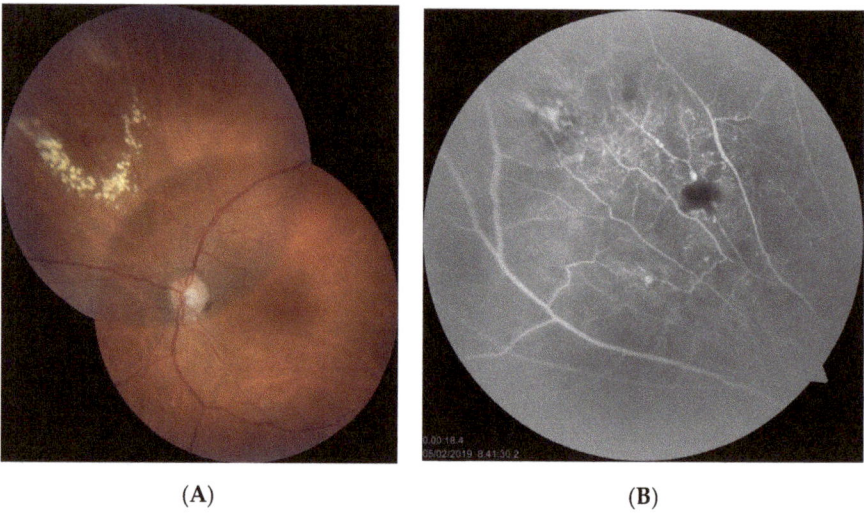

Figure 1. Fundus photograph (**A**) and FA image (**B**) of patient 2. A ring of hard exudates is visible at the periphery of the supranasal quadrant of the fundus. Fluorescein angiography revealed IPT located within the relatively small area of hard exudates. Macular edema is absent.

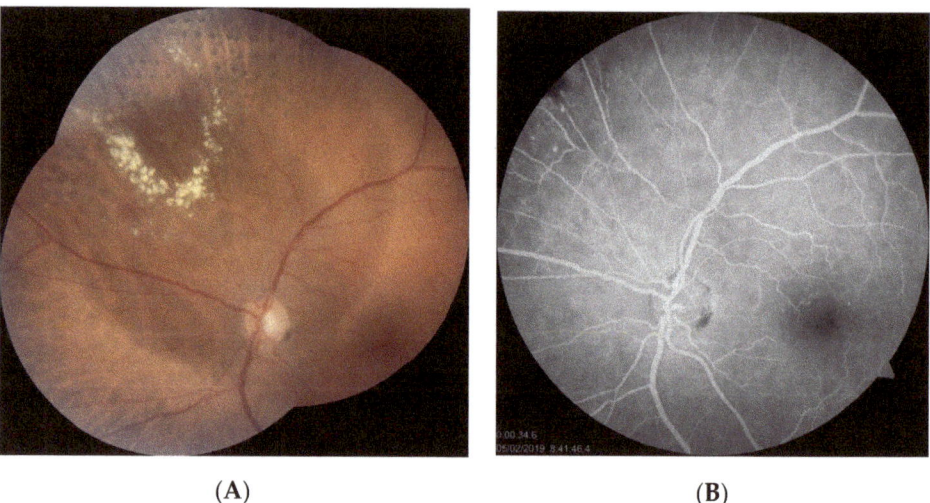

Figure 2. Fundus photograph (**A**) and FA image (**B**) of patient 2 after LPC of IPT. Partial resolution of hard exudates is visible.

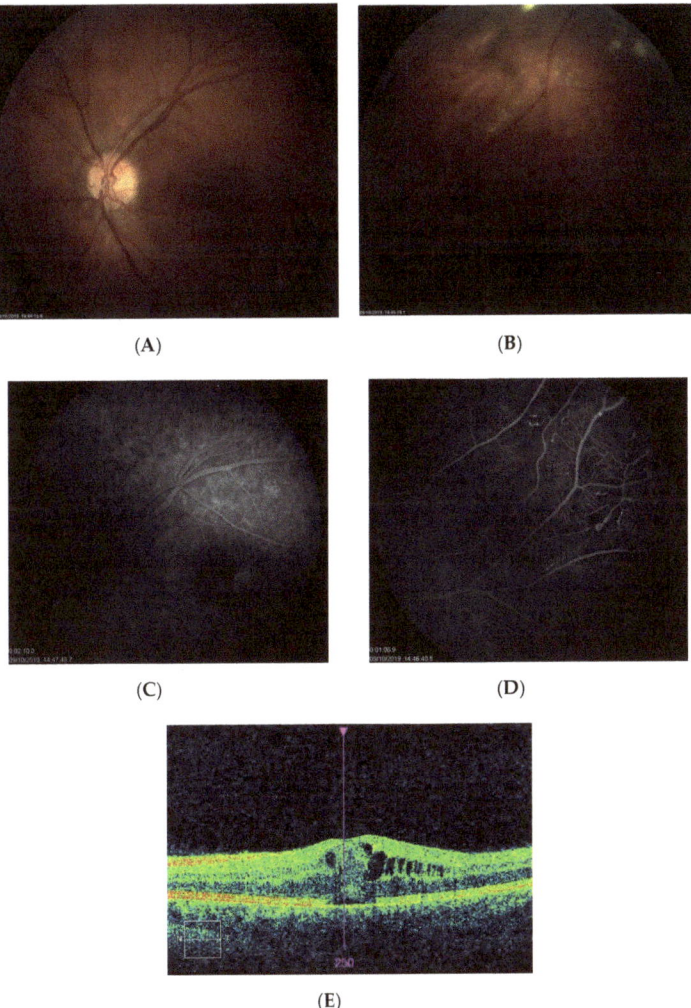

Figure 3. Pretreatment fundus photographs (**A**,**B**), FA images (**C**,**D**), and SD-OCT macular scan (**E**) of patient 3. Hard exudates are visible in supratemporal quadrant of the fundus of LE. FA reveals IPT and CME. CME is confirmed by SD-OCT scan.

Patient 4 from category 3 presented with IPT in the shape of a round, well-demarcated lesion bordering the temporal sector of the macular area and with the fovea appearing normal during the biomicroscopic examination. FA imaging revealed a typical IPT pattern within the lesion (Figure 5C). There was only a mild CME detected by SD-OCT, which was treated subsequently with subthreshold micropulse laser (Figure 5D). The patient did not show up for follow-up until his vision had significantly decreased to 20/100 at 12 months after his initial presentation. SD-OCT scan at that time revealed significant macular edema with defects at the ellipsoid zone (Figure 6A). LPC was used to create a line demarcating the lesion from the fovea in combination with intravitreal bevacizumab. Intravitreal injections were repeated several times over the following nine months, without significant morphological changes in the central retina or BCVA improvement (Figure 6B). At that point, other therapeutic options were considered, such as more intensive LPC or cryotherapy of the lesion.

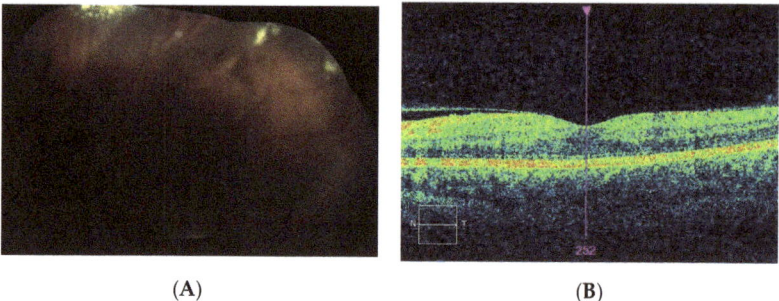

Figure 4. Fundus photograph (**A**) and SD-OCT macular scan (**B**) of patient 3 after LPC and intravitreal aflibercept therapy. Laser burns are visible on the color fundus photograph. Remission of CME is noted on the SD-OCT scans.

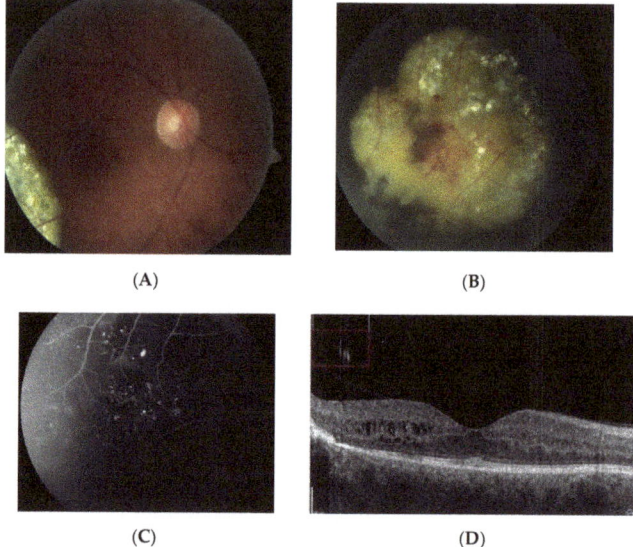

Figure 5. Fundus photographs (**A**,**B**), FA image (**C**), and SD-OCT scan (**D**) at presentation of patient 4. Color fundus photographs show a well-demarcated lesion located temporally of the macular area. FA reveals the presence of IPT within the area of the lesion. Only a mild CME is visible on the SD-OCT scan.

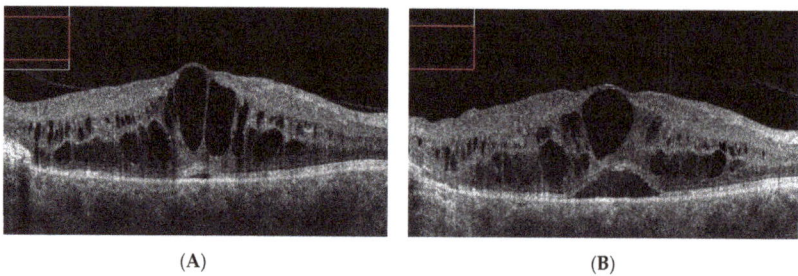

Figure 6. SD-OCT macular scans of patient 4 at 12 months after initial presentation (**A**) and after treatment with LPC and intravitreal anti-VEGF injections (**B**). Large CME with large pseudocysts is noted on the SD-OCT scans. Only a minor reduction of edema is observed after treatment.

The last patient from category 3 (patient 5) presented with a significant decrease in BCVA to 20/100. Fundus examination and FA revealed IPT in the supratemporal quadrant with an accompanying ring of hard exudates as well as CME visible on FA in the late phase (Figure 7). SD-OCT imaging confirmed the presence of significant CME with subretinal fluid and the risk of full thickness macular hole formation (Figure 7E). Vitreoretinal traction was not observed. The patient underwent LPC applied at the peripheral lesion; however, its efficacy was limited due to asteroid hyalosis, which made the procedure difficult to perform. At the moment, the patient is scheduled for supplementary LPC and intravitreal anti-VEGF treatment. Subsequent vitreoretinal surgery is also considered with increasing risk of progression to macular hole.

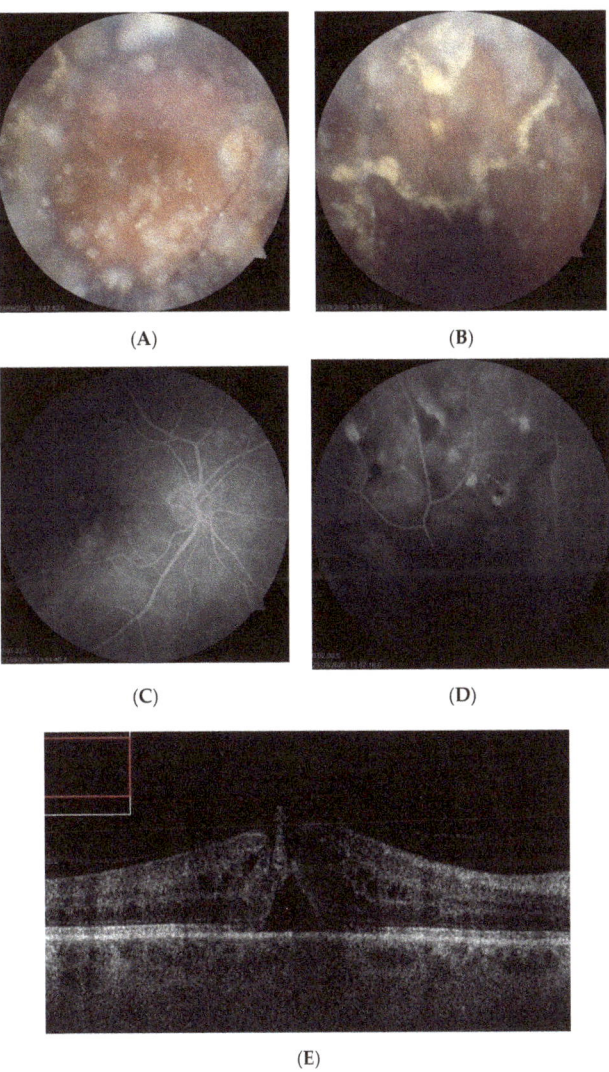

Figure 7. (**A–E**) Diagnostic images of patient 5. Fundus photographs (**A**,**B**) revealing peripheral exudates. Asteroid hyalosis obscures the visibility of the lesion. FA photos present leakage from IPT and late staining of the fovea due to CME (**C**,**D**). SD-OCT scan (**E**) confirms the presence of CME and the risk of full thickness retinal hole formation.

3.3. Category 4

One patient in group 4 was diagnosed with a significant decrease in BCVA due to macular edema with the presence of hard exudates (patient 6). The course of his disease was relatively short, in that symptoms lasted between two and three weeks. The patient was diagnosed using FA only and treated with classic LPC performed in a scatter mode at the periphery and GRID at the macula. SD-OCT and intravitreal anti-VEGF therapeutics were not present on the medical market at the time of diagnosis, so were not employed for treatment purposes. Significant functional improvement was noted one month after treatment, with further improvement in the following months. Finally, after 12 months, full central vision was restored; however, some metamorphopsia persisted. Images taken at presentation and after treatment are shown in Figures 8 and 9.

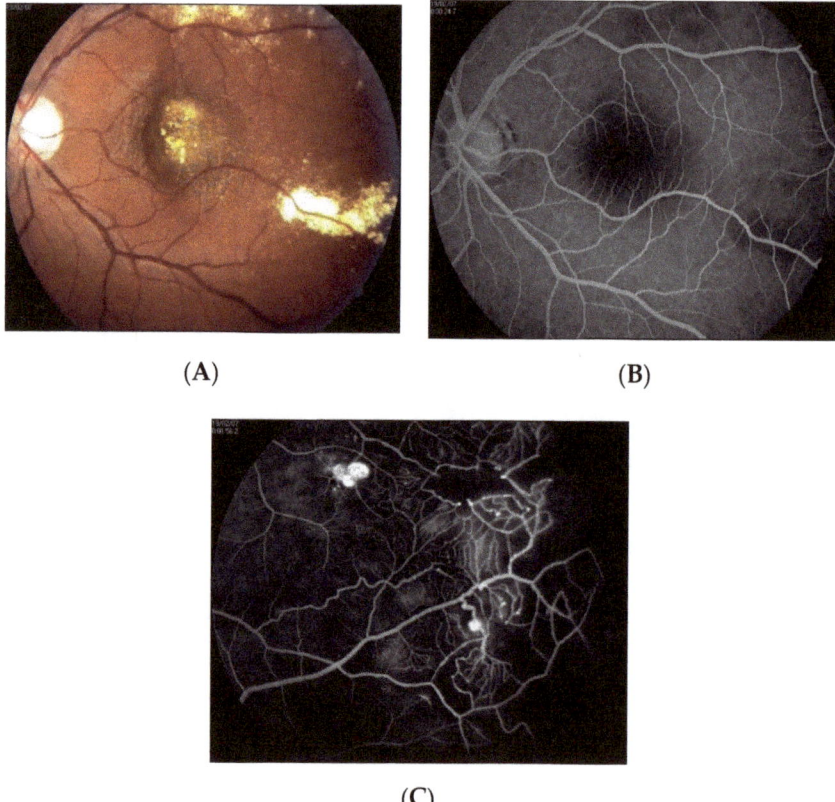

Figure 8. Fundus photographs (**A**) and FA images (**B**,**C**) at presentation of patient 6. A cluster of hard exudates is visible in the center of the macula. No vascular abnormalities were detected by FA at the fovea (**B**). Examination of the far periphery of the retina enabled visualization of large aneurysmal telangiectasias (**C**).

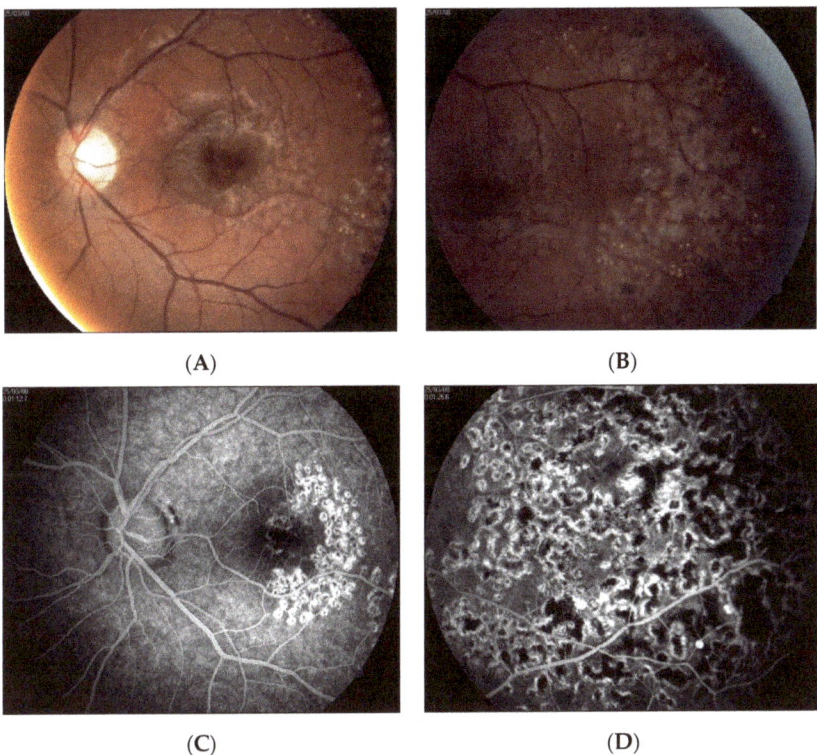

Figure 9. Patient 6 at one year after treatment. On the fundus photograph, complete resolution of hard exudates can be seen (**A**). Laser spots after GRID treatment in the macular center and after scatter photocoagulation at the periphery are noted (**B**). FA shows a lack of macular edema and destruction of the aneurysms at the periphery (**C,D**).

4. Literature Review

A literature search in PubMed for the term "peripheral retinal telangiectasias" and the combination of "Coats disease" and "adult onset" revealed 178 records, including 71 that referred to either adults only or both adults and children. Among these studies, there were 33 single case reports, 22 case reports of peripheral telangiectasia associated with systemic diseases, and 14 case series. Two reviews on wide-field diagnostics of peripheral telangiectasia were also found. Studies that reported at least three cases of adult-onset Coats disease published after 2000 were extracted and are presented in Table 3. The two largest population studies [10,15], which analyzed results of childhood and adult Coats disease in one cohort, are placed at the end of the table for reference.

Table 3. The largest adult-onset Coats disease case series, including at least three cases and reporting treatment options, published after 2000.

Study	Population	Treatment	Mean Follow-Up	Main Outcome
Smithen et al., 2005 [16]	13 adults >35 years	LPC in 11 cases; 2 cases observed (short follow-up)	5.8 years (range: 0–17)	Average loss of 2.1 lines. BCVA improvement in 2 cases, stability in 3 cases, and decline in 6 cases. At the final follow-up, BCVA ≥ 20/40 in 5 cases and BCVA < 20/200 in 3 cases.

Table 3. *Cont.*

Study	Population	Treatment	Mean Follow-Up	Main Outcome
Goel et al., 2011 [17]	3 adults	Single intravitreal bevacizumab followed by LPC	9 months	Significant improvement of BCVA in all cases of from counting fingers to 20/300, counting fingers to 20/240, and 20/240 to 20/120; regression of hard exudates from the macula in all cases
Wang et al., 2011 [18]	3 adults	2 injections of bevacizumab followed by LPC	0.5–2 years (2, 0.5, 1 years, respectively)	Significant improvement in BCVA, reduction of CRT, and regression of telangiectasias. • Case 1: BCVA change from 6/15 to 6/6.7; CRT reduction from 437 to 230 µm • Case 2: BCVA change from 6/12 to 6/6, decrease in SRF (exact numbers not reported) • Case 3: BCVA change from 5/60 to 6/20; CRT reduction from 412 to 330 µm
Zheng et al., 2014 [19]	5 adults	Intravitreal bevacizumab followed by LPC (3 cases) or intravitreal triamcinolone (1 case) or subsequent intravitreal bevacizumab (average of 2 injections during follow-up)	10.6 months	Resolution of subretinal fluid and telangiectasias without significant improvement in BCVA (range: 1.42–1.25 logMAR). Vitreoretinal fibrosis in two cases.
Park et al., 2016 [20]	13 adults	LPC combined with intravitreal bevacizumab (mean no. of injections: 2.69 and mean no of laser sessions: 1.68)	24.8 months	Mean BCVA change from 0.72 logMAR to 0.68 logMAR (statistically insignificant). BCVA improvement of more than 3 lines in 3 patients (23%) and stability in 7 patients (54%). Mean CRT was significantly decreased from 473 to 288 µm. Poor baseline BCVA and subfoveal hard exudates correlated with poor final BCVA result.
Rishi et al., 2016 [21]	48 adults ≥ 35 years 32 cases observed > 6 months	LPC (60.4%), observation (27.08%), surgery (6.2%), cryotherapy (4%), LPC plus cryotherapy (2%)	40 months (range: 1–122 months)	Patients with follow-up longer than 6 months (32 cases): • Treated: BCVA improvement or stabilization in 82.5%; exudates reduced in 56.5%, retina attached in 95.6% • Untreated: BCVA stabilization in 88%, no improvement; exudates reduced in 33%, retina attached in 66% (exact BCVA values not reported)

Table 3. Cont.

Study	Population	Treatment	Mean Follow-Up	Main Outcome
Zhang et al., 2018 [22]	12 adults	Intravitreal ranibizumab or conbercept followed by LPC	23.10 ± 7.8	Mean BCVA improvement significant from 1.27 ± 0.69 to 1.05 ± 0.73 logMAR; mean injection no. 2.33 ± 0.65, mean no. of laser treatments 2.5 ± 0.8
Reference studies: children and adults reported in one cohort				
Shields et al., 2001 [10]	124 eyes observed > 6 months Age 1 month to 63 years (average: 5 years)	Cryotherapy (42%), LPC (13%), observation (18%), surgery 17% and enucleation 11%	55 months (range: 6–300 months)	Anatomic improvement and stability in 76%. BCVA ≥ 20/50 in 14%, 20/60 to 20/100 in 6%, 20/200 to finger counting in 24%, and hand motion to light perception in 40%
Shields et al., 2019 [15]	351 cases, data from 45 years Age 0–79 years, median: 6 years	Overall (1973–2018): observation (21%), LPC (42%), cryotherapy (55%), sub-Tenon corticosteroids (12%), intravitreal corticosteroids (4%), anti-VEGF (10%), and primary enucleation (5%) Years 2010–2018: observation (11%), LPC (72%), cryotherapy (68%), sub-Tenon corticosteroids (29%), intravitreal corticosteroids (9%), anti-VEGF (18%), primary enucleation (1%)	58 months (range: 0–466 months)	BCVA overall Verbal • >20/40 (15%) • 20/50–20/200 (18%) • <20/200 (48%) Preverbal • Fix and follow (1%) • Poor fix and follow (0.4%) • No fix and follow (9%) • No cooperation (9%) BCVA Years 2010–2018 Verbal • >20/40 (24%) • 20/50–20/200 (22%) • <20/200 (40%) Preverbal • Fix and follow (1%) • Poor fix and follow (0.0%) • No fix and follow (5%) • No cooperation (6%) Disease resolution overall: 57% Disease resolution 2010–2018: 73%

BCVA—best-corrected visual acuity; CRT—central retinal thickness; LPC—laser photocoagulation; VEGF—vascular endothelial growth factor.

5. Discussion

5.1. Definitions, Classification, and Presentation

IPT (or Coats disease) falls under the umbrella of the aneurysmal form of telangiectasia potentially associated with severe intraretinal leakage, subretinal exudation, and risk of retinal detachment. This phenotype differs from MACTEL type 2, which present with small telangiectatic vessels without intraretinal leakage, typical cystic appearance of the fovea, and atrophic changes in neurosensory retina [13]. The main features of IPT are capillary, venular, and arteriolar aneurysms. If located in the macular area, these aneurysms are referred to as MACTEL type 1 and are considered by some to be a variant of Coats disease [13]. Peripheral aneurysmal telangiectasias are usually larger than macular ones and more often accompanied by areas of hypoperfusion.

The presence of peripheral telangiectasias may be correlated with some systemic disorders, some of which are very rare, and, in such cases, are not referred to as Coats disease. This is an important differentiation because it influences the choice of treatment. Peripheral telangiectasia can be found in such diseases and syndromes as aplastic anemia, Bannayan-Zonaya syndrome, cutis marmorata telangiectatica congenita, multiple sclerosis, Takayasu arteritis, Cornelia de Lange syndrome, familial exudative vitreoretinopathy, genetic myopathies, dyskeratosis congenital, Coats-like retinitis pigmentosa, and intraocular tumors [23–35].

Variable terms were used to describe IPT, especially when they occurred in adults (Table 1). Clinicians named IPT as Coats disease (or adult-onset Coats disease in older patients), Leber miliary aneurysm, or simple peripheral retinal telangiectasia. Here, the author proposes that using a single descriptive term such as "idiopathic peripheral retinal telangiectasia" or "idiopathic peripheral aneurysmal telangiectasia" would improve communication between researchers.

In this case series, adult IPT cases were categorized into four types according to patients' fundus presentation and foveal involvement. The proposed classification expands the well-established Shields categorization of early stages of Coats disease [10]. Shields categorized the presence of IPT without exudations as Stage 1 while Stage 2 included patients with IPT and extrafoveal exudations (2A) or foveal exudations (2B). The author suggests development of Shields Stage 2 into three categories, depending on the presence and severity of macular edema: IPT with peripheral exudations but without foveal involvement, IPT with peripheral exudations and cystoid macular edema but without macular exudates, and IPT with both peripheral and macular exudates and edema.

One must realize that Shields' milestone report was published in 2001 when SD-OCT and intravitreal medications were not commonly in use; instead, diagnostics in Coats disease were based on fundus examination and FA results. Nowadays, however, we are able to precisely diagnose even traceable forms of macular edema with the use of SD-OCT, which makes it possible to correlate the classification of IPT with the presence and appearance of macular edema. It must further be emphasized that cases with cystoid macular edema and a lack of central exudates can be found during the course of the disease; however, they are not specifically pointed out in the Shields classification scheme. Once they are recognized and named, it will be easier to make treatment decisions, which, in contemporary ophthalmology, involve intravitreal therapies. The four forms of presentation of patients identified in the present case series may serve as a simple alternative classification system of IPT in its mild or moderate stage without retinal detachment.

5.2. Diagnostics

Peripheral forms of retinal telangiectasia, if asymptomatic, are probably recognized and followed quite rarely. In this case series, IPT without foveal involvement were diagnosed only after very scrupulous fundus examinations. Nevertheless, these cases could have easily been omitted by other clinicians, which probably happens most of the time with asymptomatic IPT. On the other hand, symptomatic cases with macular edema require diagnostic accuracy, precision, and inquisitiveness. If the far periphery of the retina is not examined, the presence of macular edema might be attributed to a different clinical entity, such as Irving–Gass syndrome, pars planitis, diabetic retinopathy, retinal vein occlusion, or another condition (patient 3 is an example of this). The diagnostics of peripheral retinal telangiectasia are definitely easier with the use of ultra–wide-field (UWF) FA systems, which provide an easy view of the periphery of the retina [36–40]. Cases with the lesions located in the far periphery might be easily missed if only standard seven field imaging is used. UWF images can also guide treatment, as the areas of abnormal vasculature and non-perfusion are visualized more precisely [39,40]. Thus, LPC or cryotherapy in IPT cases diagnosed with UWF-FA systems are potentially more effective, as all the abnormal areas of the retina are treated. [36]. Still, the use of UWF devices is not common yet due to their high cost. Nevertheless, the analysis of diagnostic processes in IPT suggests the necessity of examining the far periphery of the retina in any case presenting with an unexplained cause of macular edema.

5.3. Treatment

Table 3 presents the results of treatment of adult cases of IPT in the largest available studies published after 2000. Visual outcomes after treatment in general were rather poor, with a minority of patients achieving final BCVA values of greater than 20/40. The introduction of intravitreal therapies and more frequent use of lasers seemed to improve visual outcomes; however, a large percentage of patients still ended up with final BCVA values below 20/200. As can be seen, material is rather scarce, so it is difficult to formulate strong treatment recommendations based solely on experience with IPT in adult cohorts. Results of treatment of Coats disease in the pediatric population should therefore also be considered while exploring the treatment of IPT in the adult population.

Category 1 and 2 in my case series, without foveal involvement, included asymptomatic patients who were referred for FA after a routine examination of the fundus. Obviously, as mentioned earlier, many IPT cases such as these can pass unrecognized until they become symptomatic. The question of whether to treat asymptomatic patients with IPT has to be asked. Shields et al., in their first large published report [10], employed observation in 100% of stage 1 cases and in 40% of stage 2 cases (the remaining 60% were treated, including 10% with LPC and 50% with cryotherapy). The authors suggested conducting observation for mild, stationary forms of IPT without exudations. A lack of exudations in general means a lack of leakage from the telangiectasias and a small risk for subretinal fluid to occur. This is why such cases can be monitored simply during regular check-ups. In this series, one patient with such a form of IPT remained under observation without conversion into the disease's exudative form.

Controversies might exist concerning cases with peripheral exudation but without macular edema. Yang et al., reported that macular disease in IPT progresses from the periphery to the center [41]. Shields et al., reported excellent visual outcomes in stage 1, but poor visual outcomes in 30% of cases in stage 2A of the disease [10]. More advanced stages of IPT involve larger disturbances of retinal morphology and are more difficult to treat. Large reports from the same center provide information on risk factors predictive of persistence of subretinal fluid despite treatment in stages 3–5 [42]. Poor outcome was associated with larger extent of telangiectasias and exudates, larger elevation of subretinal fluid, and the presence of iris neovascularization, and concerned 38% of patients. These data suggest that any case of progression or extension of leakage on the periphery should therefore be treated without delay, which can be done with the use of ablative procedures. Realistically, as peripheral LPC in adults is a rather uncomplicated and safe procedure that does not interfere with central vision, it can also be performed without waiting for documented progression of exudates.

The most challenging cases of IPT involve patients with accompanying macular edema (categories 3 and 4 in this series). The therapeutic approach in such cases has evolved since the advent of intravitreal injections; however, to date, there exist only a few studies that analyzed the efficacy of different treatment modalities solely in adults. This is probably due to the fact that, in most cases, Coats disease becomes symptomatic and is treated at younger ages. Adult-onset Coats disease is probably, as mentioned before, a milder form of its childhood variant, which appears to occur quite rarely. This is why a large number of cases are so hard to collect and contemporary treatment recommendations have to be based instead on case reports. The studies by Shields and colleagues constitute milestone reports of treatment in pediatric Coats disease. In 2001, Shields et al., listed the following therapeutic procedures applied in 150 cases of Coats disease (the authors report both childhood and adulthood cases together, with the median age of five years): observation, cryotherapy, LPC, and surgery for retinal detachment [10]. Meanwhile, the largest analysis so far (of 351 cases) treated over 45 years, also published by Shields et al., in 2019, reports a shift toward LPC and intravitreal therapies in the last 10 to 20 years [15].

The advent of anti-VEGF drugs apparently brought about a new chance for patients to achieve better functional results. It has been proven that VEGF levels are elevated in Coats disease and are related to disease severity, especially the amount of retinal exudations [43,44]. Therefore it has been suggested that the use of anti-VEGF agents promotes the absorption of exudates and a reduction in telangiectasias, thus improving functional outcomes [45].

Different anti-VEGF medications have been used in combination with ablative therapies in the treatment of Coats disease. A report from Bascom Palmer Institute details the successful treatment of 24 children with advanced Coats disease complicated by exudative retinal detachment with direct laser ablation in combination with anti-VEGF treatment [46]. Zhang et al., presented the results of 28 cases (including 12 adults) treated by the combination of LPC and intravitreal ranibizumab or conbercept [22], where LPC was applied after initial anti-VEGF injection and then both treatments were used in a pro re nata (PRN) fashion. These authors noted significant morphological improvements; however, the changes in BCVA were not statistically significant. On the other hand, Ramasubramanian and Shields warn that the addition of bevacizumab to standard Coats therapy (LPC and cryotherapy) might evoke vitreoretinal fibrosis and potentially retinal detachment, rarely seen after standard therapy [47]. However, Daruich et al., in a large pediatric study did not find such a relationship [48]. To date, this question remains unanswered, although clinicians emphasize the benefits of anti-VEGF treatment in Coats disease [17].

In this case series, two patients with IPT and macular edema were treated with the combination of intravitreal anti-VEGF and LPC and two cases were treated with LPC only. Interestingly, patient 6, after LPC monotherapy performed almost 15 years ago, practically had his BCVA completely restored, contrary to the results among patients treated after the advent of intravitreal therapies. I believe that this outcome is mainly due to the short duration of macular edema and aggressive LPC that was the treatment of choice at that time (as intravitreal injections were not available on the market yet). This is also consistent with the report by Smithen et al., from 2005, when LPC was also the main form of treatment of Coats disease in adults, where improvement or stabilization of BCVA was noted in 5 of 11 cases [16]. A large pediatric study from 2008 also reported that aggressive diode laser therapy proved effective in the majority of patients [49].

Among the remaining three cases of this series, one patient (patient 3) was treated with the combination of anti-VEGF and LPC, achieving morphological and functional success. The patient underwent very close follow-up and presented relatively early after symptoms occurred. Patient 4 after his initial visit was lost to follow-up for one year without direct aggressive laser treatment of IPT. During that time, severe macular edema developed and a decline in his BCVA to 20/200 was noted, and no improvements after combination treatment with anti-VEGF therapy plus LPC followed. I believe that the course of this case emphasizes the necessity of employing early ablative therapies in practically every case of symptomatic Coats disease. Only anecdotal reports of IPT well-controlled by anti-VEGF injections alone exist [50].

Photodynamic therapy has been trialed in the treatment of Coats disease; however, only a few case reports are available in the literature [51–53]. Thus, it should be treated as an adjunct form of treatment in refractory cases, but not as first-line therapy.

6. Conclusions

Adult-onset Coats disease is a clinical entity of variable presentation and extent. Available data support the use of ablative therapies, especially LPC, as the main and most effective means of treatment in every exudative form of peripheral telangiectasias. Only asymptomatic cases without exudates can be observed. Anti-VEGF treatment seems to be a useful adjunct to ablative therapies, especially in cases with macular involvement. Close follow-up is needed in every symptomatic adult-onset Coats disease case. Loss of follow-up without treatment might result in irreversible vision decline. Despite the application of different forms of therapies, a large percentage of adult Coats cases end up experiencing deterioration of vision and poor morphological outcomes.

Funding: No funding was received for this research.

Institutional Review Board Statement: The study was conducted according to the guidelines of the Declaration of Helsiniki and approved by the Dobry Wzrok Ophthalmological Clinic committee of EA1/2021.

Informed Consent Statement: The study was retrospective in nature and involved standard procedures performed in the clinic on a daily basis; hence, informed consent for participation in the study was waived by the Ethics Committee.

Data Availability Statement: Data is contained within the article.

Conflicts of Interest: The author declares no conflict of interest.

References

1. Coats, G. Forms of retinal diseases with massive exudation. *R. Lond. Ophthalmol. Hosp. Rep.* **1908**, *17*, 440–525.
2. Shields, J.A.; Shields, C.L.; Honavar, S.G.; Demirci, H. Clinical variations and complications of Coats disease in 150 cases: The 2000 Sanford Gifford Memorial Lecture. *Am. J. Ophthalmol.* **2001**, *131*, 561–571. [CrossRef]
3. Egbert, P.R.; Chan, C.C.; Winter, F.C. Flat preparations of the retinal vessels in Coats' disease. *J. Pediatr. Ophthalmol.* **1976**, *13*, 336–339.
4. Fernandes, B.F.; Odashiro, A.N.; Maloney, S.; Zajdenweber, M.E.; Lopes, A.G.; Burnier, M.N., Jr. Clini-cal-histopathological correlation in a case of Coats' disease. *Diagn. Pathol.* **2006**, *1*, 24. [CrossRef] [PubMed]
5. Shields, C.L.; Sen, M.; Honavar, S.G.; Shields, J.A. Coats disease: An overview of classification, management and outcomes. *Indian J. Ophthalmol.* **2019**, *67*, 763–771. [CrossRef] [PubMed]
6. Jones, J.H.; Kroll, A.J.; Lou, P.L.; Ryan, E.A. Coats' disease. *Int. Ophthalmol. Clin.* **2001**, *41*, 189–198. [CrossRef]
7. Gawecki, M. Tetniaki prosówkowate Lebera—Opis przypadku [Leber miliary aneurysms—A case report. *Klin Oczna.* **2009**, *111*, 131–133.
8. Reese, A.B. Telangiectasis of the Retina and Coats' Disease. *Am. J. Ophthalmol.* **1956**, *42*, 1–8. [CrossRef]
9. Alturkistany, W.; Waheeb, S. Leber's miliary aneurysms. *Oman J. Ophthalmol.* **2013**, *6*, 119–121. [CrossRef]
10. Shields, J.A.; Shields, C.L.; Honavar, S.G.; Demirci, H.; Cater, J. Classification and management of Coats disease: The 2000 Proctor Lecture. *Am. J. Ophthalmol.* **2001**, *131*, 572–583. [CrossRef]
11. Yanuzzi, A.L. *The Retinal Atlas*; Elsevier Ltd.: Amsterdam, The Netherlands, 2010.
12. Cahill, M.; O'Keefe, M.; Acheson, R.; Mulvihill, A.; Wallace, D.; Mooney, D. Classification of the spectrum of Coats' disease as subtypes of idiopathic retinal telangiectasis with exudation. *Acta Ophthalmol. Scand.* **2001**, *79*, 596–602. [CrossRef] [PubMed]
13. Yannuzzi, L.A.; Bardal, A.M.; Freund, K.B.; Chen, K.J.; Eandi, C.M.; Blodi, B. Idiopathic macular telangiectasia. *Arch. Ophthalmol.* **2006**, *124*, 450–460. [CrossRef] [PubMed]
14. Charbel Issa, P.; Gillies, M.C.; Chew, E.Y.; Bird, A.C.; Heeren, T.F.; Peto, T.; Holz, F.G.; Scholl, H.P. Macular telangiectasia type 2. *Prog. Retin. Eye Res.* **2013**, *34*, 49–77. [CrossRef]
15. Shields, C.L.; Udyaver, S.; Dalvin, L.A.; Lim, L.S.; Atalay, H.T.; Khoo, C.T.L.; Mazloumi, M.; Shields, J.A. Coats disease in 351 eyes: Analysis of features and outcomes over 45 years (by decade) at a single center. *Indian J. Ophthalmol.* **2019**, *67*, 772–783. [CrossRef] [PubMed]
16. Smithen, L.M.; Brown, G.C.; Brucker, A.J.; Yannuzzi, L.A.; Klais, C.M.; Spaide, R.F. Coats' Disease Diagnosed in Adulthood. *Ophthalmology* **2005**, *112*, 1072–1078. [CrossRef]
17. Goel, N.; Kumar, V.; Seth, A.; Raina, U.K.; Ghosh, B. Role of intravitreal bevacizumab in adult onset Coats' disease. *Int. Ophthalmol.* **2011**, *31*, 183–190. [CrossRef]
18. Wang, K.-Y.; Cheng, C.-K. A Combination of Intravitreal Bevacizumab Injection with Tunable Argon Yellow Laser Photocoagulation as a Treatment for Adult-Onset Coats' Disease. *J. Ocul. Pharmacol. Ther.* **2011**, *27*, 525–530. [CrossRef]
19. Zheng, X.X.; Jiang, Y.R. The effect of intravitreal bevacizumab injection as the initial treatment for Coats' disease. *Graefes Arch. Clin. Exp. Ophthalmol.* **2014**, *252*, 35–42. [CrossRef]
20. Park, S.; Cho, H.J.; Lee, D.W.; Kim, C.G.; Kim, J.W. Intravitreal bevacizumab injections combined with laser photocoagulation for adult-onset Coats' disease. *Graefe's Arch. Clin. Exp. Ophthalmol.* **2015**, *254*, 1511–1517. [CrossRef]
21. Rishi, P.; Rishi, E.; Appukuttan, B.; Uparkar, M.; Sharma, T.; Gopal, L. Coats' disease of adult-onset in 48 eyes. *Indian J. Ophthalmol.* **2016**, *64*, 518–523. [CrossRef] [PubMed]
22. Zhang, L.; Ke, Y.; Wang, W.; Shi, X.; Hei, K.; Li, X. The efficacy of conbercept or ranibizumab intravitreal injection combined with laser therapy for Coats' disease. *Graefe's Arch. Clin. Exp. Ophthalmol.* **2018**, *256*, 1339–1346. [CrossRef]
23. Metelitsina, T.I.; Sheth, V.S.; Patel, S.B.; Grassi, M.A. Peripheral retinopathy associated with aplastic anemia. *Retin. Cases Brief. Rep.* **2017**, *11*, 108–110. [CrossRef] [PubMed]
24. Klifto, M.R.; Balaratnasingam, C.; Weissman, H.H.; Yannuzzi, L.A. Bilateral coats reaction in bannayan–zonana syndrome: A single case report. *Retin. Cases Brief. Rep.* **2017**, *11*, 286–289. [CrossRef] [PubMed]
25. Taleb, E.A.; Nagpal, M.P.; Mehrotra, N.S.; Bhatt, K. Retinal findings in a case of presumed cutis marmorata telangiectatica congenita. *Retin. Cases Brief. Rep.* **2018**, *12*, 322–325. [CrossRef] [PubMed]
26. Soohoo, J.R.; McCourt, E.A.; Lenahan, D.S.; Oliver, S.C. Fluorescein angiogram findings in a case of cutis marmorata telangiectatica congenita. *Ophthalmic Surg. Lasers Imaging Retina* **2013**, *44*, 398–400. [CrossRef] [PubMed]
27. de Massougnes, S.; Borruat, F.X.; Ambresin, A. Peripheral Bilateral Telangiectasiae in Multiple Sclerosis Patients Treated with Interferon B1a. *Klin. Monbl. Augenheilkd.* **2016**, *233*, 438–440. [CrossRef] [PubMed]

28. Batliwala, S.Y.; Perez, M.; Aston, W.; Chavala, S.H. Peripheral Retinal Telangiectasia and Ischemia in Takayasu Arteritis. *Arthritis Rheumatol.* **2016**, *68*, 2350. [CrossRef]
29. Stacey, A.W.; Sparagna, C.; Borri, M.; Rizzo, S.; Hadjistilianou, T. A 6-year-old boy with Cornelia de Lange syndrome and Coats disease: Case report and review of the literature. *J. Am. Assoc. Pediatr. Ophthalmol. Strabismus* **2015**, *19*, 474–478. [CrossRef] [PubMed]
30. Ilhan, A.; Yolcu, U.; Gundogan, F.C.; Akay, F. An association between subclinical familial exudative vitreoretinopathy and rod-cone dystrophy. *Arq. Bras. Oftalmol.* **2014**, *77*. [CrossRef]
31. Kashani, A.H.; Brown, K.T.; Chang, E.; Drenser, K.A.; Capone, A.; Trese, M.T. Diversity of Retinal Vascular Anomalies in Patients with Familial Exudative Vitreoretinopathy. *Ophthalmology* **2014**, *121*, 2220–2227. [CrossRef]
32. Sacconi, S.; Baillif-Gostoli, S.; Desnuelle, C. Atteinte rétinienne et myopathies génétiques [Retinal involvement and genetic myopathy]. *Rev. Neurol.* **2010**, *166*, 998–1009. [CrossRef]
33. Johnson, C.A.; Hatfield, M.; Pulido, J.S. Retinal vasculopathy in a family with autosomal dominant dyskeratosis congenita. *Ophthalmic Genet.* **2009**, *30*, 181–184. [CrossRef] [PubMed]
34. Kan, E.; Yilmaz, T.; Aydemir, O.; Güler, M.; Kurt, J. Coats-like retinitis pigmentosa: Reports of three cases. *Clin. Ophthalmol.* **2007**, *1*, 193–198. [PubMed]
35. Char, D.H. Coats' syndrome: Long term follow up. *Br. J. Ophthalmol.* **2000**, *84*, 37–39. [CrossRef]
36. Kumar, V.; Chandra, P.; Kumar, A. Ultra-wide field imaging in the diagnosis and management of adult-onset Coats' disease. *Clin. Exp. Optom.* **2017**, *100*, 79–82. [CrossRef] [PubMed]
37. Joussen, A.M.; Brockmann, C.; Urban, J.; Seibel, I.; Winterhalter, S.; Zeitz, O.; Müller, B. Ultraweitwinkel-Fundusfotografie und -angiografie in der Differenzialdiagnose und zur Therapieplanung bei peripheren vaskulären Netzhauterkrankungen [Ultra-Wide Field Retinal Imaging and Angiography in the Differential Diagnosis and Therapeutic Decisions in Vascular Diseases of the Peripheral Retina]. *Klin. Monbl. Augenheilkd.* **2018**, *235*, 980–993.
38. Sakurada, Y.; Freund, K.B.; Yannuzzi, L.A. Multimodal Imaging in Adult-Onset Coats' Disease. *Ophthalmology* **2018**, *125*, 485. [CrossRef]
39. Temkar, S.; Azad, S.V.; Chawla, R.; Damodaran, S.; Garg, G.; Regani, H.; Nawazish, S.; Raj, N.; Venkatraman, V. Ultra-widefield fundus fluorescein angiography in pediatric retinal vascular diseases. *Indian J. Ophthalmol.* **2019**, *67*, 788–794. [CrossRef]
40. Turczyńska, M.; Brydak-Godowska, J. The role of peripheral retinal angiography in the diagnosis of adult Coats' disease based on a case report. *Klin. Ocz.* **2020**, *122*, 171–176. [CrossRef]
41. Yang, L.-H.; Shi, X.-H.; Tian, B.; Zhou, D.; Wei, W.-B. Clinical analysis of macular disease involved by Coats disease. *[Zhonghua yan ke za zhi] Chin. J. Ophthalmol.* **2009**, *45*.
42. Khoo, C.T.L.; Dalvin, L.A.; Lim, L.S.; Mazloumi, M.; Atalay, H.T.; Udyaver, S.; Shields, J.A.; Shields, C.L. Fac-tors Predictive of Subretinal Fluid Resolution in Coats Disease: Analysis of 177 Eyes in 177 Pa-tients at a Single Center. *Asia Pac. J. Ophthalmol.* **2019**, *8*, 290–297. [CrossRef]
43. Zhao, Q.; Peng, X.-Y.; Chen, F.-H.; Zhang, Y.-P.; Wang, L.; You, Q.-S.; Jonas, J.B. Vascular endothelial growth factor in Coats' disease. *Acta Ophthalmol.* **2013**, *92*, e225–e228. [CrossRef] [PubMed]
44. Zhang, J.; Jiang, C.; Ruan, L.; Huang, X. Associations of cytokine concentrations in aqueous humour with retinal vascular abnormalities and exudation in Coats' disease. *Acta Ophthalmol.* **2019**, *97*, 319–324. [CrossRef]
45. Yang, Q.; Wei, W.; Shi, X. Successful use of intravitreal ranibizumab injection and combined treatment in the management of Coats' disease. *Acta Ophthalmol.* **2016**, *94*, 401–406. [CrossRef] [PubMed]
46. Gold, A.S.; Villegas, V.M.; Murray, T.G.; Berrocal, A.M. Advanced Coats' disease treated with intravitreal bevacizumab combined with laser vascular ablation. *Clin. Ophthalmol.* **2014**, *8*, 973–976. [CrossRef]
47. Ramasubramanian, A.; Shields, C.L. Bevacizumab for Coats' disease with exudative retinal detachment and risk of vitreoretinal traction. *Br. J. Ophthalmol.* **2011**, *96*, 356–359. [CrossRef] [PubMed]
48. Daruich, A.; Matet, A.; Tran, H.V.; Gaillard, M.-C.; Munier, F.L. Extramacular fibrosis in coats' disease. *Retina* **2016**, *36*, 2022–2028. [CrossRef]
49. Schefler, A.C.; Berrocal, A.M.; Murray, T.G. Advanced Coats' disease. Management with repetitive aggressive laser ablation therapy. *Retina* **2008**, *28* (Suppl. 3), S38–S41. [CrossRef]
50. Georgakopoulos, C.D.; Foteini, T.; Makri, O.E.; Vavvas, D. Two-year results of intravitreal injections of aflibercept in Coats' Disease; a case report. *Retin. Cases Brief. Rep.* **2020**. [CrossRef]
51. Beselga, D.; Campos, A.; Mendes, S.; Carvalheira, F.; Castro, M.; Castanheira, D. Refractory Coats' Disease of Adult Onset. *Case Rep. Ophthalmol.* **2012**, *3*, 118–122. [CrossRef]
52. Namba, M.; Shiode, Y.; Morizane, Y.; Kimura, S.; Hosokawa, M.; Doi, S.; Toshima, S.; Takahashi, K.; Hosogi, M.; Fujiwara, A.; et al. Successful resolution of coats disease by photodynamic therapy: A case report. *BMC Ophthalmol.* **2018**, *18*, 264. [CrossRef] [PubMed]
53. Kim, J.; Park, K.H.; Woo, S.J. Combined Photodynamic Therapy and Intravitreal Bevacizumab Injection for the Treatment of Adult Coats' Disease: A Case Report. *Korean J. Ophthalmol.* **2010**, *24*, 374–376. [CrossRef] [PubMed]

Article

Bleb Compressive Sutures in the Management of Hypotony Maculopathy after Glaucoma Surgery

Ewa Kosior-Jarecka [1,*], Dominika Wróbel-Dudzińska [1], Anna Święch [2] and Tomasz Żarnowski [1]

1 Department of Diagnostics and Microsurgery of Glaucoma, Medical University of Lublin, 20-059 Lublin, Poland; dwrobeldudzinska@interia.pl (D.W.-D.); zarnowskit@poczta.onet.pl (T.Ż.)
2 Department of Vitreoretinal Surgery, Medical University of Lublin, 20-059 Lublin, Poland; anna.zub@umlub.pl
* Correspondence: ewakosiorjarecka@umlub.pl

Abstract: PURPOSE: The aim of the study was to assess the efficacy and safety of compressive sutures in patients with hypotony maculopathy after glaucoma surgery. METHODS: This retrospective case series analyzes the clinical outcomes of conjunctival compressive sutures in 17 patients with hypotony maculopathy developed after glaucoma surgery. Compressive Nylon 10–0 single sutures were used in all patients; in two patients, the procedure was repeated. All patients underwent ophthalmic evaluation and macular OCT scanning before the surgery, one month, six months, and one year after the procedure. RESULTS: Mean intraocular pressure (IOP) before suturing was 2.3 ± 1.57 mmHg and increased to 14.2 ± 7.03 mmHg ($p = 0.00065$) one month after the procedure. After six months, mean IOP was 10.2 ± 4.3 mmHg ($p = 0.005$), and after one year ± 4.7 mmHg ($p = 0.0117$). To obtain the target pressure, the sutures had to be removed in one patient, and medical therapy was undertaken in three patients. Mean decimal best-corrected visual acuity (BCVA) before the sutures was 0.18 ± 0.13 and increased to 0.53 ± 0.25 ($p = 0.0004$) after one month, to 0.46 ± 0.31 ($p = 0.005$) after six months, and to 0.31 ± 0.22 ($p = 0.025$) after one year. In one case, leakage from the bleb was observed after the procedure and bleb revision was required. CONCLUSIONS: transconjuctival compressive sutures seem to be an efficient and safe technique for managing hypotony maculopathy after glaucoma surgery.

Keywords: hypotony maculopathy; complications of antiglaucoma surgery; bleb compressive sutures

1. Introduction

Glaucoma, one of the leading causes of irreversible blindness worldwide [1], is a progressive optic neuropathy, and elevated intraocular pressure (IOP) is one of the main risk factors for the development and progression of this disease [2]. A decrease of IOP remains the only clinical method with confirmed efficacy for diminishing the progression rate of glaucoma, and this effect can be achieved by means of medical treatment, laser, or surgery [3].

After trabeculectomy, a standard surgical glaucoma procedure, aqueous humor flows into the surgically created filtering bleb [4]. The final success of trabeculectomy depends not only on the surgical technique but also on the possibility of slowing down the healing processes [5]. Therefore, the challenge faced by both surgical technique and postsurgical care is to find a balance between IOP low enough to obtain the target pressure and at the same time high enough to avoid complications related to ocular hypotony [6]. Additionally, not every case of post-surgical low IOP level leads to ocular complications [7].

Clinical hypotony is defined as a level of IOP that is too low to maintain the shape of the eyeball and results in structural and functional changes [8,9]. If left untreated, prolonged hypotony may cause various serious complications such as bleb infection, cataract formation, synechiae, persistent choroidal detachment, or hypotony maculopathy [10]. Hypotony maculopathy and bleb infection in the course of clinical hypotony are potentially sight-threatening [11,12].

The clinical characteristics of hypotony maculopathy were first described by Dellaporta in 1954 as "creasing of retina in hypotonia" [13], but the modern definition of hypotony maculopathy was introduced by Gass to emphasize the etiology of vision loss in the setting of chorioretinal folds [14]. Macular hypotony is characterized by a decrease in visual acuity caused by macular folds, retinal edema, papilledema, and vascular tortuosity. Structurally, it is believed that low IOP level causes thickening of the perifoveal choroid and sclera, which results in their central displacement, visible as macular folds. Over time, these changes cause photoreceptor damage and become irreversible, which can limit recovery of visual function even after restoration of normal IOP [15,16].

Treatment options for hypotony after glaucoma surgery mainly caused by overfiltrating blebs include conservative management of topical autologous serum [17], bleb injection of autologous blood [18] or viscoelastic material [19], and anterior chamber injection of viscoelastic material [20] or gas [21]. Conservative management usually has minor and only short-lasting effects. Surgical management includes transconjunctival flap suturing [22,23], excision of thin blebs and conjunctival advancement [16], patch grafting using donor sclera [24,25], donor cornea [26], and autologous conjunctiva [27,28]. The variety of described techniques shows that all these procedures have their disadvantages. On the other hand, the techniques that reduce the transscleral flow by suturing or tissue patching may lead to limitation of the outflow resulting in very high IOP elevation [29].

Transconjunctival compressive sutures were introduced to the management of postsurgical hypotony as a simple and effective technique [30]. The aim of the study was to evaluate the efficacy and safety of transconjunctival suturing of overfiltrating blebs in hypotony maculopathy after glaucoma surgery.

2. Materials and Methods

The studied group consisted of 17 Caucasian patients with hypotony maculopathy after glaucoma surgery treated in the Department of Diagnostics and Microsurgery of Glaucoma, Medical University of Lublin, Poland, between 2015 and 2017. During this period, every patient who met inclusion criteria participated in the study.

The inclusion criteria was as follows:
- Age at glaucoma diagnosis of over 18 years;
- At least 6 months after the antiglaucoma procedure;
- Clinically significant hypotony: intraocular pressure (IOP) lower than 6 mmHg, associated with the BCVA decreased by at least 2 lines on Snellen charts in comparison to pre-trabeculectomy results;
- Features of hypotony maculopathy with macular folds;
- No progression of the cataract;
- No leakage from the bleb;
- No kissing choroidal effusion.

Clinical and demographic characteristics of the studied group are presented in Table 1. The studied group included 7 patients with primary open angle glaucoma (POAG), 4 with glaucoma in the course of pigment dispersion syndrome (PDSG), 4 with pseudo-exfoliative glaucoma (PEXG) and 1 with primary angle closure glaucoma (PACG).

Table 1. Clinical and demographic characteristics of the studied group.

Feature	n/Mean Value ± SD
Number of patients	17
Gender	8F/10 M
Age	60.5 ± 20.5
Diagnosis	POAG: 7 cases; PDSG: 4 cases: PEXG: 4 cases; PACG: 1 case; traumatic glaucoma: 1 case.
Primary procedure	Trabeculectomy: 9 cases; Phacotrabeculectomy: 4 cases; Needle revision: 3 cases; Deep sclerectomy: 1 case.
Mean IOP before primary procedure	33.6 ± 11.6 mmHg
Mean IOP before sutures	2.3 ± 1.57 mmHg
BCVA before primary procedure	0.55 ± 0.31
BCVA before sutures	0.18 ± 0.13
Mean MD	16.21 ± 7.45 dB
Mean time between primary procedure and compression sutures	3.08 years

POAG, primary open angle glaucoma; PDSG, pigment dispersion syndrome; PEXG, pseudo-exfoliative glaucoma; PACG, primary angle closure glaucoma; IOP, mean intraocular pressure; BCVA, best-corrected visual acuity; MD, mean deviation.

The information about patients' medical history was obtained from their clinical records. At the inclusion visit, patients underwent ophthalmic examination with BCVA (decimal Snellen charts), Goldman applanation tonometry, slit lamp examination, eye fundus assessment by ophthalmoscopy, and OCT (Stratus, Carl Zeiss Meditec, Dublin, Ireland) measurements assessing the thickness of the macula and the presence of choroidal folds.

During the surgical procedure, 5–7 single Nylon 10–0 sutures were placed transconjunctivally in the area of the bleb as described earlier [30]. In brief, after peribulbar anesthesia, the bulb was rotated downward and single sutures were placed, starting from the limbus and extending posteriorly as far as possible toward the superior fornix. During suturing, attempts were made to catch not only the conjunctiva but also a part of the underlying sclera, if the height of the bleb allowed for it. The sutures were intended to be placed on the area of existing scleral flap or in its proximity. During the procedure, after placing the 5th suture, paracentesis was performed and the BSS was administered into the anterior chamber to assess the increase of IOP and the reduction of the outflow. Further sutures were added until the increase in IOP was observed (up to 7 sutures). The idea and the surgical technique are shown in Scheme 1.

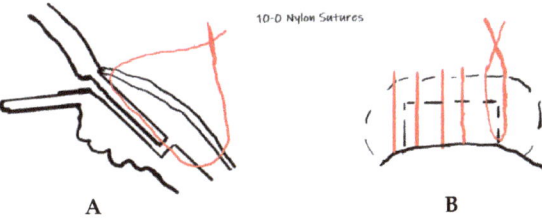

Scheme 1. Transconjunctival sutures placement: **A**, side view; **B**, front view.

In the post-surgical period, only fixed combination of dexamethasone/tobramycine was used in decreasing doses (starting from 4 times a day, and decreasing 1 drop per week up to 4 weeks when the drops were stopped). Some patients needed to have installed the preservatives free lubricant drops.

The patients were controlled one day after the procedure, as well as 7 days, 1 month, 3 months, 6 months, and 12 months after the procedure. During the check-ups, ophthalmic examination was performed including BCVA testing (decimal Snellen charts), Goldman applanation tonometry, slit lamp examination, eye fundus assessment by ophthalmoscopy, and OCT measurements assessing the thickness of the macula and the presence of choroidal folds. All patients were present at all time-point visits. However, in 2 cases at 6 months, OCT was not performed because of technical problems. Additionally, the study eye was examined at every visit to look for possible complications.

Two criteria of success were defined:
1. IOP over 6 mmHg;
2. BCVA improvement of at least 2 lines on a Snellen chart.

Changes in the assessed values (BCVA and IOP) were measured at each control visit planned in the study by subtracting the preoperative value from the postoperative value. Statistic evaluation of the data was performed using Statistica 13.1 (Polish version, Statsoft Poland). The results were reported mainly as mean ± SD or percentage values. A p-value lower than 0.05 was considered statistically significant. Normal distribution was assessed with the Shapiro–Wilk test. The Mann–Whitney test was used for non-normally distributed data.

3. Results

Mean IOP before suturing was 2.3 ± 1.57 mmHg and increased to 14.2 ± 7.03 mmHg ($p = 0.00065$) at 1 month post-op. After 6 months, mean IOP was 10.2 ± 4.3 mmHg ($p = 0.005$); and after one year ± 4.7 mmHg ($p = 0.0117$) (Figure 1). On day 7 after surgery, IOP value exceeded 21 mmHg in 4 (23.5%) patients, with a value of over 30 mmHg in one case. To obtain the target pressure, one patient needed to have one suture removed, and medical therapy was undertaken in three patients.

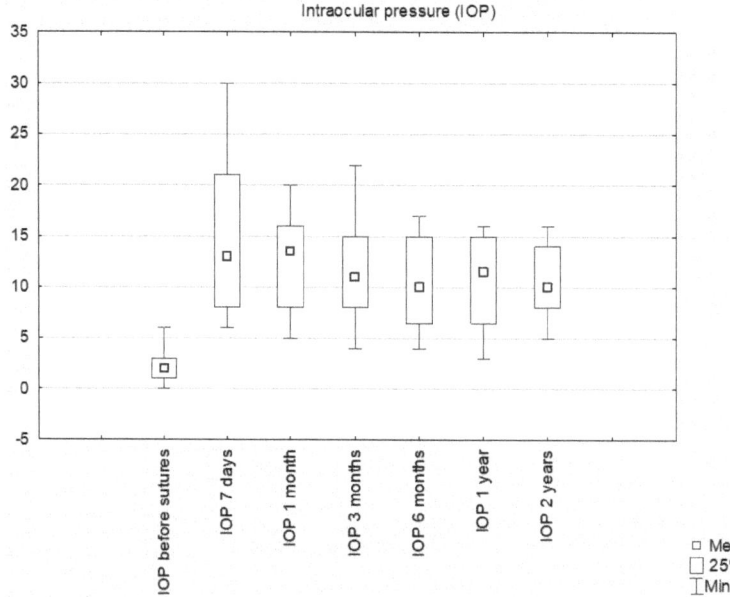

Figure 1. Changes in the intraocular pressure during the study period.

Success criterion 1 (IOP over 6 mmHg) at 7 days post-procedure was achieved in 15 (88%) patients, after 3 months in 10 (59%) patients, and after 6 months in 9 (53%) patients (and remained stable during the first and second year of follow-up).

Mean BCVA before applying the sutures was 0.18 ± 0.13 and increased to 0.53 ± 0.25 ($p = 0.0004$) after 1 month; to 0.46 ± 0.31 ($p = 0.005$) after 6 months; and to 0.31 ± 0.22 ($p = 0.025$) after one year (Figure 2).

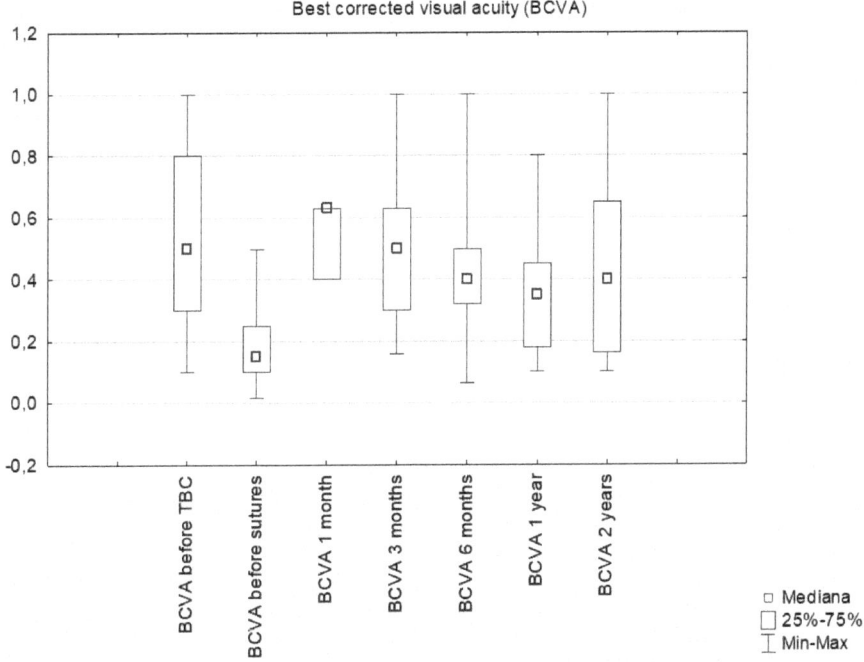

Figure 2. Changes in best-corrected visual acuity during the study period.

Success Criterion 2 (BCVA improvement of at least 2 lines) was fulfilled in the whole studied group at 3 months post-procedure, in 14 patients (82%) at 6 months, in 12 (71%) at 1 year, and in 11 (65%) at 2 years.

Mean subfoveal macular thickness before suturing was 316.33 μm, and decreased to 283.22 μm at 1 month ($p = 0.0314$), and to 279.77 μm at 1 year ($p = 0.0322$) (Figure 3). Macular folds were present in every patients at the inclusion. Starting from 3rd month macular folds were not observed during ophthalmoscopy in 7 patients (41.1%).

No significant correlations were found between the change in IOP and the change in mean subfoveal macular thickness in OCT, except for the tendency to a negative correlation between these results obtained at 6 months ($p = 0.1050$; $R = -0.61$). Interestingly, we could not find any significant correlations between the change in macular thickness in OCT and the change in BCVA ($p = 0.9329$ at 3 months; $p = 0.2682$ at 6 months, and 0.644512 at 1 year).

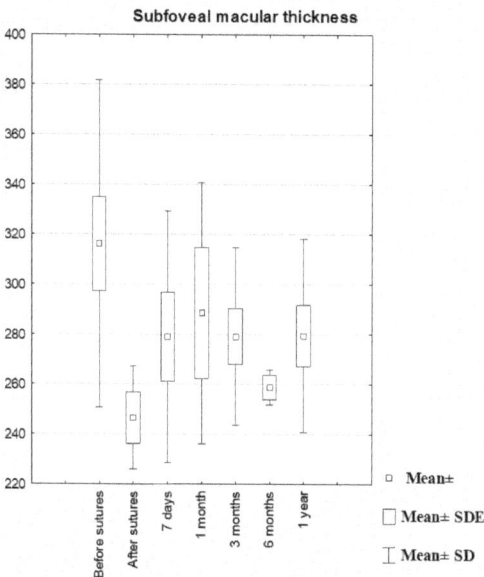

Figure 3. Changes in the subfoveal macular thickness assessed by optical coherent tomography during the study period.

The mean time between the primary surgery and compression suturing was 3.08 years. The time between the primary surgery and suturing did not correlate with postoperative IOP ($p = 0.9537$ at 1 month; $p = 0.5181$ at 3 months, $p = 0.2333$ at 6 months, and $p = 0.6895$ at 1 year). Assessing the influence of the time since the primary procedure on the final BCVA, we observed negative tendencies at 3 and 6 months ($p = 0.2725$, $R = -0.34$, and $p = 0.1553$, $R = -0.51$, respectively) and a significant negative correlation at 1 year ($p = 0.0138$; $R = -0.94$).

When our group was divided into 2 subgroups: with time from the primary surgery shorter than one year (early group: 8 patients) and longer than a year (late group: 9 patients), no differences in BCVA were found (late: 0.18 vs. early: 0.16, $p = 0.2470$ before sutures; late: 0.33 vs. early: 0.37, $p = 0.7881$ at 1 year). The initial IOP did not differ the groups (late: 1.67 mmHg vs. early: 2.65 mmHg; $p = 0.3799$). However, the IOP seemed to be higher in early group with statistical tendency at 1 year (late: 7.33 mmHg vs. early: 11.78; $p = 0.1671$) and statistical significance at 2 years (late: 6.66 mmHg vs. early: 12.5 mmHg; $p = 0.0067$).

Two patients had peripheral choroidal detachments at the inclusion, which resolved within 7 days post-op. In one case, leakage from the bleb was observed after the procedure, and bleb revision procedure was needed.

The exemplary case is presented on Figure 4.

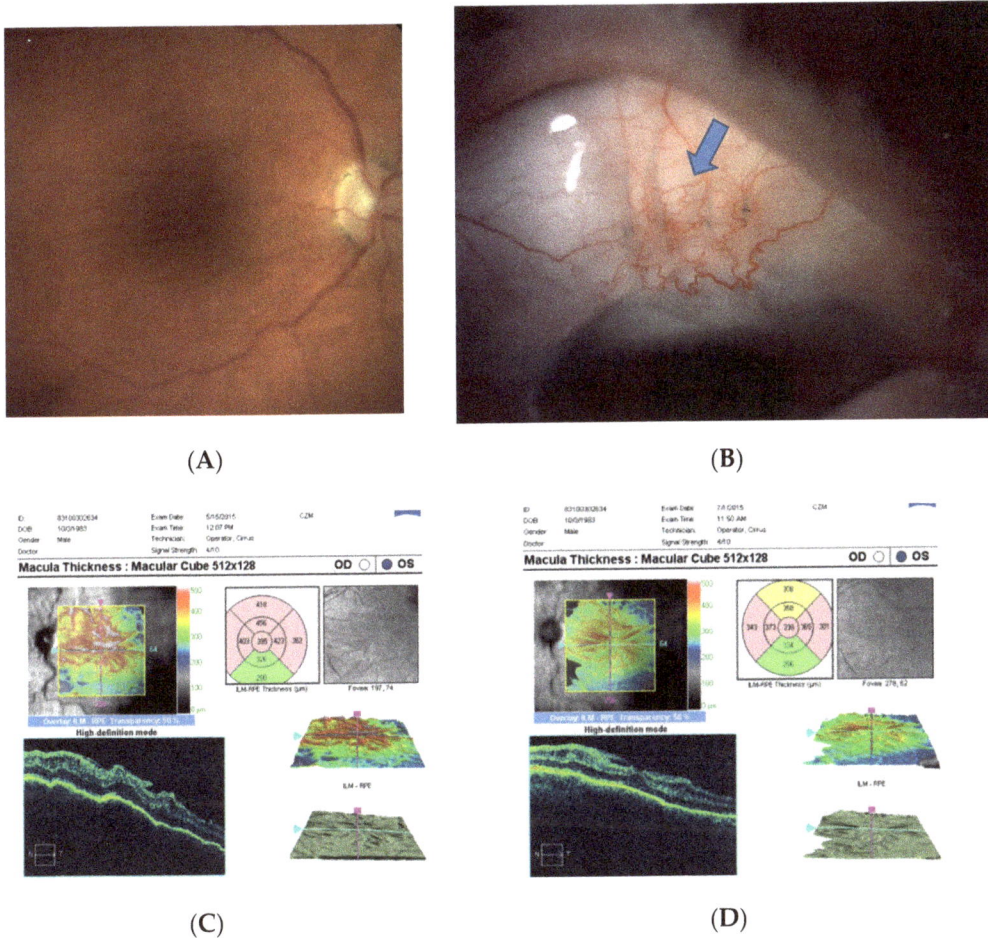

Figure 4. Sample case. (**A**) Eye fundus with hypotony maculopathy; (**B**) compressive sutures—1 day after the surgery (blue arrow points the sutures); (**C**) macular OCT before suturing; (**D**) macular OCT after suturing.

4. Discussion

The wide range of reported chronic hypotony after antiglaucoma procedures is due to the lack of a standardized definition [31,32]. Additionally, some eyes require very low IOP to stop or slow down glaucoma progression [33]. In cases when pre-surgery IOP has lower values or when glaucomatous optic neuropathy is advanced, an IOP below 6 mm Hg without cataract progression, choroidal effusion, or maculopathy, and with improved glaucoma is considered a surgical success [34]. In this study, transconjunctival suturing was performed when the IOP maintained under 6 mmHg and the BCVA remained significantly decreased due to hypotony maculopathy.

The perfect time for intervention in case of hypotony after antiglaucoma procedure is also not clear. The tendency to delay the treatment is observed because clinical experience suggests that most eyes with chronic hypotony following a trabeculectomy maintain good visual acuity without complications [11]. Moreover, spontaneous recovery from hypotony caused by natural healing processes is frequent [34]. Additionally, a lot of procedures designed to cure hypotony turn out to be unsuccessful: 5 of our patients had previously had blood injected to the bleb to enhance healing without prolonged effect.

The duration of hypotony has been reported to have no correlation with final visual outcomes [11,35]. In the case of our patients with hypotony maculopathy, we observed that the time since the primary procedure indeed did not influence the final IOP level after transconjunctival suturing. If timely managed, IOP increase usually leads to the restoration of the normal smooth architecture of the retina, allowing for realignment of photoreceptors and visual recovery [31]. On the other hand, prolonged hypotony causes irreversible fibrosis within the retina, choroid, or sclera, maintaining the choroid in a folded position [31]. Scoralick et al. found resolution of hypotony maculopathy in 85% of the cases following surgical reintervention, but none of the variables investigated (including the time interval between trabeculectomy and flap resuturing) was significantly associated with postoperative maculopathy resolution [36].

Numerous risk factors for hypotony after glaucoma surgery have been identified, including myopia, young age, antimetabolite use, pre-existing inflammation, aphakia, and old age accompanied by a thin conjunctiva and thinner CCT [11,37,38]. Besides the application of an antifibrotic agent, male gender, high myopia, young age, and patients receiving primary filtering surgery have also been associated with an increased risk of hypotony maculopathy [39,40]. In our study, five (29%) patients underwent primary procedure at the age below 40 because of pigmentary glaucoma or traumatic glaucoma. It confirms the susceptibility of younger patients to hypotony maculopathy. Additionally, all of these patients were myopic males, which suggests that care needs to be taken in this group during the primary procedure to avoid hypotony, with lower titers of antimetabolites and tight bleb suturing. Lower scleral rigidity in younger patients is believed to be related to the development of hypotony maculopathy [14,40]. Additionally, myopic eyes tend to have thinner sclera, which is related to a general loss of collagen and proteoglycans [41] and makes sclera more vulnerable to collapse during hypotony. Further, males tend to have lower scleral rigidity and a correlation between male gender and hypotony maculopathy has been ascertained [42].

In our practice, transconjunctival sutures are an effective and safe method of increasing IOP and improving visual acuity in patients with hypotony maculopathy as a complication of antiglaucoma procedure. In a retrospective study, Letarte et al. showed a significant IOP increase and BCVA improvement six months after transconjunctival scleral flap resuturing [43]. Eha et al. [22,44] published a prospective case study describing the outcome of 16 patients whose mean IOP was 9.6 mmHg and mean BCVA was 20/60, six months following the procedure. These results are similar to ours with mean IOP value of 9 mmHg 1 year after suturing. We observed a gradual decrease in mean IOP in the course of the study, with the highest values one month postoperatively.

Although the success in IOP increase was not observed in every patient, during the early postoperative period we observed an improvement of the visual acuity in the whole group, similarly to the results observed by Scoralick [36]. It shows the efficacy of transconjunctival sutures regarding BCVA improvement, and probably additionally confirms that numerous definitions of hypotony are not accurate, as in some patients an increase in IOP even below 6 mmHg allowed for BCVA improvement.

In our group, but not in every case, it was possible to obtain the stable IOP increase in post-surgical period, which may have some possible reasons. First, it may be connected with not enough traction obtained during placement of the sutures, which is usually connected with the changes of the ocular tissues during early postsurgical period (for example, the decrease in conjunctival oedema or moving of the sutures through the conjunctiva). Tight suturing with the attachment to the superficial parts of the sclera in case of extensively hyperfiltarating and elevated blebs may also be problematic. Additionally, it is possible that after MMC application during primary procedure the scleral tissues are weakened and melted which makes transconjunctival suturing not enough for limitation of the outflow. In such cases, the revision with opening of conjunctiva and direct suturing of the sclera may be beneficial. Finally, after antiglaucoma procedure prolonged ciliary body hypoperfusion and hyposecretion is possible.

Clinical assessment had led us to the assumption that a shorter time since the primary procedure may enable obtaining a more prominent increase in the IOP level, which was not confirmed by our results: in this study, at no time-point was IOP correlated with the time since the primary surgery, which was also observed by other authors [36]. However, in our results a longer time since the primary surgery tended to have a negative impact on the final BCVA. It may be related to the observation that when left untreated, hypotony maculopathy can have long-term visual consequences [7] with irreversible chorioretinal folds resulting from fibrosis within the retina, choroids, or sclera [31,45]. Additionally, in our study the patients with sutures placed earlier tended to have higher IOP values in longer observation period. This is why our results may provide an argument for an earlier intervention in maculopathy hypotony. However, in our opinion, the surprising finding of this study is the lack of correlation between the improvement in BCVA and the changes in subfoveal macular thickness determined in OCT. It may be explained by the fact that during the study, intra- or sub-retinal fluid was not observed; thus, the initial BCVA decrease after the antiglaucoma procedure was not caused by any disturbances in the morphology of the retinal layers but rather by their folding. Additionally, the improvement in BCVA may be partially explained by the restoration of the anterior segment structures after the increase in IOP [46–48]. The changes in the hemodynamics of the choroid affected by the IOP increase may also be involved in BCVA improvement [49].

In general, the highest IOP during the follow-up period was measured on postoperative Day 7. Furthermore, this spike in IOP seemed to be beneficial for expediting the resolution of any preexisting serous choroidal detachments [16] and cause quicker improvement in BCVA, as observed in this study. However, in such cases, the improvement of the visual acuity was not stable; all three patients with the decrease in BCVA observed at six months belonged to this group. The highest values of early postoperative IOP were observed in the group of younger patients with pigmentary glaucoma, which may also be connected with scleral vulnerability, as mentioned earlier. On the other hand, such high spikes in IOP may be potentially harmful in the case of severely damaged visual field in advanced glaucoma.

Except for the observed IOP spikes, transconjunctival sutures seem to be a safe procedure. In the course of the study, we observed only one patient with avascular thin bleb who suffered from bleb leakage and needed bleb revision, which involved covering it with the mobilized conjunctiva.

To sum up, transconjunctival sutures seem to be an effective and safe method to treat hypotony maculopathy after glaucoma surgery. In the study, the improvement in BCVA started with the elevation of IOP at the early postoperative period and remained stable during the observation time. Our results also provide an argument for an earlier intervention in case of clinical hypotony after glaucoma surgery.

Author Contributions: Conceptualization, E.K.-J. and T.Ż.; methodology, E.K.-J. and T.Ż.; software, D.W.-D.; formal analysis, E.K.-J. and D.W.-D.; investigation, E.K.-J., D.W.-D and A.Ś.; resources T.Ż.; data curation D.W.-D.; writing—original draft preparation E.K.-J.; writing—review and editing, E.K.-J., D.W.-D., A.Ś. and T.Ż.; supervision, T.Ż. All authors have read and agreed to the published version of the manuscript.

Funding: This research received no external funding.

Institutional Review Board Statement: The study was conducted according to the guidelines of the Declaration of Helsinki, and approved by the Local Board of Ethics Committee of Medical University of Lublin (Approval nr127/2015).

Informed Consent Statement: Informed consent was obtained from all subjects involved in the study.

Data Availability Statement: Data are available from the corresponding author on demand.

Conflicts of Interest: The authors declare no conflict of interest.

References

1. Quigley, H.A.; Broman, A.T. The number of people with glaucoma worldwide in 2010 and 2020. *Br. J. Ophthalmol.* **2006**, *90*, 262–267. [CrossRef] [PubMed]
2. Weinreb, R.N.; Aung, T.; Medeiros, F.A. The pathophysiology and treatment of glaucoma: A review. *JAMA* **2014**, *14*, 1901–1911. [CrossRef]
3. Weinreb, R.N.; Khaw, P.T. Primary open-angle glaucoma. *Lancet* **2004**, *22*, 1711–1720. [CrossRef]
4. Khaw, P.T.; Chiang, M.; Shah, P.; Sii, F.; Lockwood, A.; Khalili, A. Enhanced Trabeculectomy: The Moorfields Safer Surgery System. *Dev. Ophthalmol.* **2017**, *59*, 15–35. [CrossRef] [PubMed]
5. Joseph, J.P.; Miller, M.H.; Hitchings, R.A. Wound healing as a barrier to successful filtration surgery. *Eye* **1988**, *2*, S113–S123. [CrossRef]
6. Costa, V.P.; Arcieri, E.S. Hypotony maculopathy. *Acta Ophthalmol. Scand.* **2007**, *85*, 586–597. [CrossRef] [PubMed]
7. Seah, S.K.; Prata, J.A., Jr.; Minckler, D.S.; Baerveldt, G.; Lee, P.P.; Heuer, D.K. Hypotony following trabeculectomy. *J. Glaucoma* **1995**, *4*, 73–79. [CrossRef]
8. Pederson, J.E. Ocular Hypotony. In *The Glaucomas*; Ritch, R., Krupin, T., Shields, M.B., Eds.; Mosby: St. Louis, MO, USA, 1996; pp. 385–395.
9. Rahman, A.; Mendonca, M.; Simmons, R.B.; Simmons, R.J. Hypotony after glaucoma filtration surgery. *Int. Ophthalmol. Clin.* **2000**, *40*, 127–136. [CrossRef]
10. Edmunds, B.; Thompson, J.R.; Salmon, J.F.; Wormald, R.P. The National Survey of Trabeculectomy. III. Early and late complications. *Eye* **2002**, *16*, 297–303. [CrossRef]
11. Saeedi, O.J.; Jefferys, J.L.; Solus, J.F.; Jampel, H.D.; Quigley, H.A. Risk factors for adverse consequences of low intraocular pressure after trabeculectomy. *J. Glaucoma* **2014**, *23*, e60–e68. [CrossRef]
12. Francis, B.A.; Hong, B.; Winarko, J.; Kawji, S.; Dustin, L.; Chopra, V. Vision loss and recovery after trabeculectomy: Risk and associated risk factors. *Arch. Ophthalmol.* **2011**, *129*, 1011–1017. [CrossRef] [PubMed]
13. Dellaporta, A. Creasing of retina in hypotonia. *Klin. Mon. Augenheilkd. Augenarztl. Fortbild.* **1954**, *125*, 872–878.
14. Gass, J.D. Hypotony Maculopathy. In *Contemporary Ophthalmology: Honoring Sir Stewart Duke-Elder*; Bellows, J.G., Ed.; Williams and Wilkins: Baltimore, MD, USA, 1972; pp. 336–343.
15. Oyakhire, J.O.; Moroi, S.E. Clinical and anatomical reversal of long-term hypotony maculopathy. *Am. J. Ophthalmol.* **2004**, *137*, 953–995. [CrossRef] [PubMed]
16. Bitrian, E.; Song, B.J.; Caprioli, J. Bleb revision for resolution of hypotony maculopathy following primary trabeculectomy. *Am. J. Ophthalmol.* **2014**, *158*, 597–604.e1. [CrossRef] [PubMed]
17. Matsuo, H.; Tomidokoro, A.; Tomita, G.; Araie, M. Topical application of autologous serum for the treatment of lateonset aqueous oozing or point-leak through filtering bleb. *Eye* **2005**, *19*, 23–28. [CrossRef] [PubMed]
18. Smith, M.F.; Magauran, R.G., 3rd; Betchkal, J.; Doyle, J.W. Treatment of postfiltration bleb leaks with autologous blood. *Ophthalmology* **1995**, *102*, 868–871. [CrossRef]
19. Higashide, T.; Tagawa, S.; Sugiyama, K. Intraoperative Healon5 injection into blebs for small conjunctival breaks created during trabeculectomy. *J. Cataract Refract. Surg.* **2005**, *31*, 1279–1282. [CrossRef]
20. Hosoda, S.; Yuki, K.; Ono, T.; Tsubota, K. Ophthalmic viscoelastic device injection for the treatment of flat anterior chamber after trabeculectomy: A case series study. *Clin. Ophthalmol.* **2013**, *7*, 1781–1785.
21. Kurtz, S.; Leibovitch, I. Combined perfluoropropane gas and viscoelastic material injection for anterior chamber reformation following trabeculectomy. *Br. J. Ophthalmol.* **2002**, *86*, 1225–1227. [CrossRef]
22. Eha, J.; Hoffmann, E.M.; Wahl, J.; Pfeiffer, N. Flap suture—A simple technique for the revision of hypotony maculopathy following trabeculectomy with mitomycin C. *Graefes Arch. Clin. Exp. Ophthalmol.* **2008**, *246*, 869–874. [CrossRef]
23. Shirato, S.; Maruyama, K.; Haneda, M. Resuturing the sclera flap through conjunctiva for treatment of excess filtration. *Am. J. Ophthalmol.* **2004**, *137*, 173–174. [CrossRef] [PubMed]
24. Haynes, W.L.; Alward, W.L. Rapid visual recovery and longterm intraocular pressure control after donor scleral patch grafting for trabeculectomy-induced hypotony maculopathy. *J. Glaucoma* **1995**, *4*, 200–201. [CrossRef] [PubMed]
25. Harizman, N.; Ben-Cnaan, R.; Goldenfeld, M.; Levkovitch-Verbin, H.; Melamed, S. Donor scleral patch for treating hypotony due to leaking and/or overfiltering blebs. *J. Glaucoma* **2005**, *14*, 492–496. [CrossRef] [PubMed]
26. Bochmann, F.; Kaufmann, C.; Kipfer, A.; Thiel, M.A. Corneal patch graft for the repair of late-onset hypotony or filtering bleb leak after trabeculectomy: A new surgical technique. *J. Glaucoma* **2014**, *23*, e76–e80. [CrossRef] [PubMed]
27. Panday, M.; Shantha, B.; George, R.; Boda, S.; Vijaya, L. Outcomes of bleb excision with free autologous conjunctival patch grafting for bleb leak and hypotony after glaucoma filtering surgery. *J. Glaucoma* **2011**, *20*, 392–397. [CrossRef] [PubMed]
28. Dietlein, T.S.; Lappas, A.; Rosentreter, A. Secondary subconjunctival implantation of a biodegradable collagen-glycosaminoglycan matrix to treat ocular hypotony following trabeculectomy with mitomycin C. *Br. J. Ophthalmol.* **2013**, *97*, 985–988. [CrossRef]
29. Laspas, P.; Wahl, J.; Peters, H.; Prokosch-Willing, V.; Chronopoulos, P.; Grehn, F.; Pfeiffer, N.; Hoffmann, E.M. Outcome of Bleb Revision With Autologous Conjunctival Graft Alone or Combined With Donor Scleral Graft for Late-onset Bleb Leakage with Hypotony after Standard Trabeculectomy with Mitomycin C. *J. Glaucoma* **2021**, *1*, 175–179. [CrossRef]

30. Maruyama, K.; Shirato, S. Efficacy and safety of transconjunctival scleral flap resuturing for hypotony after glaucoma filtering surgery. *Graefes Arch. Clin. Exp. Ophthalmol.* **2008**, *246*, 1751–1756. [CrossRef]
31. Jampel, H.D.; Pasquale, L.R.; Dibernardo, C. Hypotony maculopathy following trabeculectomy with mitomycin C. *Arch. Ophthalmol.* **1992**, *110*, 1049–1050. [CrossRef]
32. Thomas, M.; Vajaranant, T.S.; Aref, A.A. Hypotony maculopathy: Clinical presentation and therapeutic methods. *Ophthalmol. Ther.* **2015**, *4*, 79–88. [CrossRef]
33. Higashide, T.; Ohkubo, S.; Sugimoto, Y.; Kiuchi, Y.; Sugiyama, K. Persistent hypotony after trabeculectomy: Incidence and associated factors in the Collaborative Bleb-Related Infection Incidence and Treatment Study. *Jpn. J. Ophthalmol.* **2016**, *60*, 309–318. [CrossRef] [PubMed]
34. Yun, S.; Chua, B.; Clement, C.I. Does Chronic Hypotony following Trabeculectomy Represent Treatment Failure? *J. Curr. Glaucoma Pract.* **2015**, *9*, 12–15. [CrossRef] [PubMed]
35. Cohen, S.M.; Flynn, H.W., Jr.; Palmberg, P.F.; Gass, J.D.; Grajewski, A.L.; Parrish, R.K., 2nd. Treatment of hypotony maculopathy after trabeculectomy. *Ophthalmic Surg. Lasers* **1995**, *26*, 435–441. [CrossRef] [PubMed]
36. Scoralick, A.L.B.; Almeida, I.; Ushida, M.; Dias, D.T.; Dorairaj, S.; Prata, T.S.; Kanadani, F.N. Hypotony Management through Transconjunctival Scleral Flap Resuturing: Analysis of Surgical Outcomes and Success Predictors. *J. Curr. Glaucoma Pract.* **2017**, *11*, 58–62. [CrossRef] [PubMed]
37. Stamper, R. Bilateral chronic hypotony following trabeculectomy with mitomycin C. *J. Glaucoma* **2001**, *10*, 325–328. [CrossRef]
38. Silva, R.A.; Doshi, A.; Law, S.K.; Singh, K. Postfiltration hypotony maculopathy in young chinese myopic women with glaucomatous appearing optic neuropathy. *J. Glaucoma* **2010**, *19*, 105–110. [CrossRef]
39. Singh, K.; Byrd, S.; Egbert, P.R.; Budenz, D. Risk of hypotony after primary trabeculectomy with antifibrotic agents in a black West African population. *J. Glaucoma* **1998**, *7*, 82–85. [CrossRef]
40. Fannin, L.A.; Schiffman, J.C.; Budenz, D.L. Risk factors for hypotony maculopathy. *Ophthalmology* **2003**, *110*, 1185–1191. [CrossRef]
41. Curtin, B.J.; Iwamoto, T.; Renaldo, D.P. Normal and staphylomatous sclera of high myopia. An electron microscopic study. *Arch. Ophthalmol.* **1979**, *97*, 912–915. [CrossRef]
42. Nicolela, M.T.; Carrillo, M.M.; Yan, D.B.; Rafuse, P.E. Relationship between central corneal thickness and hypotony maculo-pathy after trabeculectomy. *Ophthalmology* **2007**, *114*, 1266–1271. [CrossRef] [PubMed]
43. Letartre, L.; Basheikh, A.; Anctil, J.-L.; Des Marchais, B.; Goyette, A.; Kasner, O.P.; Lajoie, C. Transconjunctival suturing of the scleral flap for overfiltration with hypotony maculopathy after trabeculectomy. *Can. J. Ophthalmol.* **2009**, *44*, 567–570. [CrossRef] [PubMed]
44. Eha, J.; Hoffmann, E.M.; Pfeiffer, N. Long-term results after transconjunctival resuturing of the scleral flap in hypotony following trabeculectomy. *Am. J. Ophthalmol.* **2013**, *155*, 864–869. [CrossRef] [PubMed]
45. Tunç, Y.; Tetikoglu, M.; Kara, N.; Sagdık, H.M.; Özarpaci, S.; Elçioğlu, M.N. Management of hypotony and flat anterior chamber associated with glaucoma filtration surgery. *Int. J. Ophthalmol.* **2015**, *8*, 950–953.
46. Cashwell, L.F.; Martin, C.A. Axial length decrease accompanying successful glaucoma filtration surgery. *Ophthalmology* **1999**, *106*, 2307–2311. [CrossRef]
47. Camp, A.S.; Weinreb, R.N. Hypotony Keratopathy Following Trabeculectomy. *J. Glaucoma* **2020**, *29*, 77–80. [CrossRef] [PubMed]
48. Azuma, K.; Saito, H.; Takao, M.; Araie, M. Frequency of hypotonic maculopathy observed by spectral domain optical coherence tomography in post glaucoma filtration surgery eyes. *Am. J. Ophthalmol. Case Rep.* **2020**, *18*, 100786. [CrossRef] [PubMed]
49. Saeedi, O.; Pillar, A.; Jefferys, J.; Arora, K.; Friedman, D.; Quigley, H. Change in choroidal thickness and axial length with change in intraocular pressure after trabeculectomy. *Br. J. Ophthalmol.* **2014**, *98*, 976–979. [CrossRef]

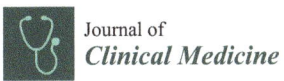

Article

Dysregulated Tear Film Proteins in Macular Edema Due to the Neovascular Age-Related Macular Degeneration Are Involved in the Regulation of Protein Clearance, Inflammation, and Neovascularization

Mateusz Winiarczyk [1,*], Dagmara Winiarczyk [2], Katarzyna Michalak [2], Kai Kaarniranta [3], Łukasz Adaszek [2], Stanisław Winiarczyk [2] and Jerzy Mackiewicz [1]

1. Department of Vitreoretinal Surgery, Medical University of Lublin, 20-079 Lublin, Poland; jerzymackiewicz@umlub.pl
2. Department of Epizootiology, University of Life Sciences of Lublin, 20-400 Lublin, Poland; winiarczykdm@gmail.com (D.W.); artica@wp.pl (K.M.); lukasz.adaszek@up.lublin.pl (Ł.A.); genp53@interia.pl (S.W.)
3. Department of Ophthalmology, University of Eastern Finland and Kuopio University Hospital, 70211 Kuopio, Finland; kai.kaarniranta@uef.fi
* Correspondence: mateuszwiniarczyk@umlub.pl; Tel.: +48-692-476-464

Abstract: Macular edema and its further complications due to the leakage from the choroidal neovascularization in course of the age-related macular degeneration (AMD) is a leading cause of blindness among elderly individuals in developed countries. Changes in tear film proteomic composition have been reported to occur in various ophthalmic and systemic diseases. There is an evidence that the acute form of neovascular AMD may be reflected in the tear film composition. Tear film was collected with Schirmer strips from patients with neovascular AMD and sex- and age-matched control patients. Two-dimensional electrophoresis was performed followed by MALDI-TOF mass spectrometry for identification of differentially expressed proteins. Quantitative analysis of the differential electrophoretic spots was performed with Delta2D software. Altogether, 11 significantly differentially expressed proteins were identified; of those, 8 were downregulated, and 3 were upregulated in the tear film of neovascular AMD patients. The differentially expressed proteins identified in tear film were involved in signaling pathways associated with impaired protein clearance, persistent inflammation, and neovascularization. Tear film protein analysis is a novel way to screen AMD-related biomarkers.

Keywords: age-related macular degeneration; AMD; proteomics; tear film; tear film proteome; protein clearance; neovascularization; neovascular AMD

1. Introduction

Age-related macular degeneration (AMD) is a leading cause of blindness in elderly patients in developed countries. The incidence of AMD is expected to increase by over 50% in the next 20 years [1]. AMD affects central vision by evoking metamorphopsia, reading problems, and eventually legal blindness in its end stage. AMD can be divided into wet (neovascular) and dry (atrophic) forms. Usually, atrophic AMD progresses slowly over years, while neovascular AMD with the presence of subretinal fluid and macular edema can develop in weeks due to the progressive growth of pathological choroidal vessels. Currently, there is no established treatment protocol for atrophic AMD, but anti-vascular endothelial growth factor (VEGF) intravitreal injections are a treatment of choice for neovascular AMD. Although our awareness of AMD etiopathology has significantly improved in the past decade, the exact mechanisms underlying the disease are still vague. The cellular mechanisms of AMD are known to be linked to chronic oxidative stress (OS), autophagy impairment, and inflammation that can ultimately lead to retinal pigment epithelium (RPE) cell and photoreceptor death [2,3]. AMD development is also strongly associated with genetic variations and mutations in the complement system, as well as with many environmental risk factors, such as smoking, hypercholesterolemia, arteriosclerosis, obesity, and unhealthy diet consumption [4].

Tear film is a mixture of lipids, water, and mucin that covers the surface of the eye. It protects against an environment-evoked irritation and smooths the corneal surface to improve the refractive effect. Tear film is produced by lacrimal and accessory glands, as well as by meibomian glands and goblet cells [5]. Since tear film is readily accessible, it has been analyzed in many clinical studies on dry eye syndrome, diabetes, Parkinson's disease, multiple sclerosis, and cancer [6–12].

Previous studies concerning proteomic changes that occur over the course of AMD have focused mainly on the aqueous humor, the vitreous body, donor retinas, and blood [13–29]. In each of these studies, significant differences in the expression of certain proteins have been discovered. The identified proteins are usually involved in metabolic pathways associated with AMD. We reviewed most of the recent developments in AMD proteomic research in our previous manuscript, in which we sought to determine whether the pathological process in the macula can result in tear film proteome changes [30]. Although we discovered various differentially expressed proteins, we were not able to perform quantitative analysis. In this study, we analyzed tear film samples from neovascular AMD patients to identify and quantify proteins that were differentially expressed between a neovascular AMD group and a control group.

2. Materials and Methods

The study was approved by the Bioethical Committee of the Medical University of Lublin under declaration number KE-0254/238/2015. Informed consent was obtained from every individual enrolled in the study. The purpose and design of the study, as well as its possible complications, were explained to every patient, and written consent was obtained. All experiments followed the provisions of the Declaration of Helsinki.

In total, 30 patients were included in the study: 15 patients in the neovascular AMD group, and 15 in the control group. The sex distribution was similar between the groups. All criteria-satisfying patients underwent a full ophthalmic examination by the same ophthalmologist (MW) that consisted of a visual acuity test, slit lamp examination, intraocular pressure (IOP) measurement, spectral domain optical coherent tomography (SDOCT, Copernicus, Optopol Technologies, Zawiercie, Poland), and fluorescein angiography or optical coherence tomography angiography (angio-OCT, RTVue XR 100 Avanti, Optovue, Fremont, CA, USA). The tear film break-up times (BUTs) were within normal limits (over 10 s), and all the patients had Schirmer test results of greater than 15 mm in 5 min.

The inclusion criteria for the AMD group were as follows: active form of disease featuring choroidal neovascularization (CNV) on fluorescein angiography or angio-OCT in at least one eye and the presence of subretinal fluid.

The exclusion criteria were any ocular surface diseases that would disturb the results, e.g., dry eye syndrome, eye surface disorders, diabetic retinopathy, glaucoma, and previous ocular surgery except for cataract extraction. Additionally, any moderately advanced or advanced stage of any systemic disease, such as poorly controlled hypertension, cardiovascular disease, or autoimmune disorder, was an exclusion criterion.

The neovascular AMD group consisted of 15 patients, comprising 7 men and 8 women, with a mean age of 76.4 years (SD = 5.6). On slit lamp examination, the patients presented with an active form of AMD in at least one eye with subretinal fluid presence. All of them had previously been treated with anti-VEGF therapy in one or both eyes. Environmental risk factors, smoking, and systemic diseases were assessed. The control subjects were recruited from among patients who qualified for standard cataract surgery. The control group consisted of 15 patients, comprising 8 men and 7 women, with a mean age of 76.1 years (SD = 3.9). The mean IOP was within normal limits (8–21 mm Hg) in all patients.

For a statistical analysis of sex difference, a chi-square test on the contingency table with control and AMD on one side and male and female on the other side, making a 2 × 2 table, and assuming the null hypothesis about independence of health from gender. Comparing the chi-square-calculated parameter with the tabular value, we dealt with independent variables, meaning that the gender composition of the groups was neutral. According to the age comparison between the groups, we performed a t-test to determine the difference in the means. In this case (group one mean: 76.4 ± 5.4; group two: 76.1 ± 3.9), the p-value equals 0.8782. By conventional criteria, this difference is not considered to be statistically significant. To confirm that the groups were statistically similar, we preformed the Shapiro–Wilk test of normality. We accepted that H0 assumed that the data in the control and AMD groups were normally distributed. We also accepted H0 in the t-test, which meant that the average of 1's population was considered to be equal to the average of the 2's population. In other words, the difference between the average of the 1 and 2 populations was not big enough to be statistically significant.

Detailed information about the study and the control groups are presented in Supplementary Materials Tables S1 and S2.

2.1. Sample Preparation

Tear film was collected from each eye onto a Schirmer strip (TearFlo, HUB Pharmaceuticals LLC, Scottsdale, AZ, USA) [1,2]. Each collection was performed by the author M.W. in the morning hours between 8 and 11 a.m. If fluorescein angiography was performed, the material was always collected beforehand. Sterile gloves were always used by the investigator. The Schirmer strips were placed into the lower conjunctival sacs of both eyes at the one-third point of the eyelid as measured from the nasal canthus without anesthesia. There is currently no consensus about which method of collection should be used for proteomic analysis [3–6]. After the strips were held in place for 5 min, they were removed, transferred to 1.5-mL Eppendorf tubes without buffer, and immediately frozen at −80 °C. Next, the proteins were extracted in urea buffer for 3 h. Extraction was carried out at 4 °C in the presence of protease inhibitor cocktail (P8340, Sigma Aldrich, St. Louis, MO, USA). The cocktail contained 104 mM 4-(2-aminoethyl)benzenesulfonyl fluoride hydrochloride (AEBSF), 80 μM aprotinin, 4 mM bestatin, 1.4 mM E-64, 2 mM leupeptin, and 1.5 mM pepstatin A. Each of these components has specific inhibitory properties. AEBSF and aprotinin inhibit serine proteases, including trypsin, chymotrypsin, and plasmin, among others; bestatin inhibits aminopeptidases; E-64 inhibits cysteine proteases; leupeptin inhibits both serine and cysteine proteases; and pepstatin A inhibits acid proteases (according to the Sigma–Aldrich specification sheet). After extraction, the strips were removed, and the extracts were centrifuged at 1844× g for 10 min at 4 °C. The obtained supernatants were collected and stored at −80 °C.

2.2. Protein Purification and Precipitation

The concentrations of the proteins were measured by a spectrophotometric method (MaestroNano Micro-Volume Spectrophotometer). Samples containing 150 μg of proteins were transferred into 1.5-mL microcentrifuge tubes and diluted with water to a final volume of 100 μL. Using a ReadyPrep 2-D Cleanup Kit (Bio-Rad, Hercules, CA, USA) the protein pellets were obtained and resuspended by adding 300 μL of rehydration sample buffer (Bio-Rad). The supernatants were applied directly to immobilized pH gradient (IPG) strips (17 cm, pH 3¨C10, linear pH gradient, Bio-Rad).

After 12 h of gel rehydration the isoelectric focusing was performed at 60 kVh with a current limit of 50 μA per strip (Hoefer IEF100). Before second-dimension separation, the IPG strips were equilibrated in two equilibration buffers (50 mM Tris-HCl, pH 8.8, 6 M urea, 30% glycerol, 2% sodium dodecyl sulfate (SDS)). The first buffer contained dithiothreitol (2%), while the second buffer contained iodoacetamide (2.5%) instead of dithiothreitol. The duration of each equilibration step was 15 min. The second dimension of electrophoretic separation was conducted using 12.5% polyacrylamide gels in a Bio-Rad PROTEAN II xi Cell (Bio-Rad). Vertical separation was performed at 600 V/50 mA/30 W in 0.025 M Tris/Gly buffer (pH 8.3). After electrophoretic separation, the proteins were silver stained in accordance with the methods of Shevchenko et al. [7].

2.3. Preparation of Proteins for MALDI Identification

The spots of interest were excised from the gels by scalpel, transferred into microtubes, washed with H_2O, and distained. After that, dithiothreitol reduction and iodoacetamide alkylation were performed. The gel pieces were covered with trypsin solution containing 50 mM ammonium bicarbonate and placed in an autoclave overnight to digest at 37 °C. Next, the peptides were extracted from the gel pieces with 50 µL of acetonitrile (ACN):H_2O:trifluoroacetic acid (TFA) (50:45:5) solution. Extraction was performed in an ultrasonic bath at room temperature and was repeated three times (each step lasted 15 min). The extracts were collected and concentrated in a CentriVap (Labconco, Kansas City, MO, USA). The obtained peptide pellets were dissolved in 10 µL of 0.1% TFA and purified with ZipTip Sample Prep Pipette Tips (0.2 µL of C18 iod, Merck, Darmstadt, Germany) in accordance with a standard procedure.

2.4. MALDI Analysis

Finally, 1 µL of each purified peptide sample was spotted onto an AnchorChip MALDI plate with hydrophobic coating and calibrant anchors. Next, 1 µL of alpha-cyano-4-hydroxycinnamic acid (HCCA, Bruker, Billerica, MA, USA) matrix solution was pipetted onto the dry peptide sample. A peptide calibration standard (Peptide Calibration Standard II, Bruker) was spotted on the calibrant spots. The mass spectra were recorded in active positive reflection mode by an Ultraflex III MALDI-TOF/TOF spectrometer (Bruker). All spectra were collected within the 700–4000 m/z range. The collected spectra were smoothed (Savitsky–Golay method) and the baseline corrected (Top Hat baseline algorithm) in flexAnalysis 3.0 software (Bruker). A list of peaks in the range of 700–4000 m/z for a signal-to-noise ratio greater than 3 was also generated in flexAnalysis 3.0. After removal of impurities, the final peak list was transferred to BioTools 3.2 (Bruker) and compared with Mascot 2.2 software using the Swiss–Prot database. Other parameters were set as follows: the maximum error in both MS and MS/MS was 0.3 Da; the obligatory modification was carbamidomethylation of cysteine; and the possible modifications were methionine oxidation, serine, and threonine phosphorylation, methionine dioxidation, and protein N-terminal acetylation. Results with scores above 56 were considered statistically significant. The peptide mass fingerprint spectra were analyzed in MS/MS mode to confirm the amino acid sequences.

2.5. Visual and Statistical Analysis

The stained gels were scanned using a GE Image Scanner III (GE Healthcare, Warsaw, Poland) and further processed by Delta2D software (version 4.7, DECODON). The Delta2D software enabled quantitation of the spots and creation of protein expression profiles. The utilized program uses gel image warping (correction of positional spot variations and matching of images) to create a so-called fused image. This image is a proteome map containing every protein spot obtained on every gel during the whole experiment. After the fused image was created, the spots were detected. False-negative and false-positive protein spots were determined manually. To calculate the expression ratios (Rts; spot volumes relative to the group means), a quantitation table was generated, and the volume-normalized values were statistically analyzed. In this experiment, the mean volume of a given spot in the control group was the denominator of the Rt parameter.

In the case of gel statistical analysis after normalization, we used a *t*-test for two analyzed groups with *p*-values based on t-distribution and alpha (overall all threshold *p*-value): 0.05. We took a Rt value greater than 1.5 as overexpressed and below 0.67 as suppressed.

Differences in protein expression between the test groups were analyzed by a t-test with statistical software built into Delta2D; a p-value ≤ 0.05 was considered to indicate significance. The p-value of 0.05 was two-sided ($\alpha/2 = 0.025$ both sides). Only spots with significant differential expression between the neovascular AMD group and the control group, and with spot Rts higher than 1.5 (upregulated) or lower than 0.67 (downregulated), were selected for protein identification.

3. Results

Altogether, samples from 15 patients with neovascular AMD and 15 control patients were included in the proteomic analysis. Differences in protein expression levels between the two groups were identified using two-dimensional gel electrophoresis (2DE) followed by MALDI-TOF MS.

We chose groups to be as similar to each other as possible in terms of age, disease, and gender. In the AMD group, the mean age was 76.4 years $\pm$ 5.4. Patients who took part in the study were mostly smokers (73%) with systemic diseases (40% had one disease, 33% had two). This group of 15 patients consisted of 7 men (47%) and 8 females (53%). The control group was similar: The mean age was 76.1 $\pm$ 3.8, and 73% were also smokers. When it comes to the occurrence of systematic diseases, the numbers are also analogous: 40% had one disease, 33% had two. There was a minimal sex difference: the control group of 15 individuals consisted of 8 men (53%) and 7 females (47%).

We found 469 proteins in the analyzed tear film samples. Among those, we focused only on the differential electrophoretic spots. Bioanalytical software revealed that 31 spots exhibited significant differences between groups, and 14 spots fulfilled the Rt criteria of greater than 1.5 (upregulated) or less than 0.67 (downregulated), in three consecutive repetitions. Fourteen of the spots were positively identified. From those, 11 proteins were eventually identified, as Annexin A1 was recognized 3 times, and Retinal dehydrogenase twice. The same proteins occurring in different points of gel is a common finding. Spot multiplicity is mostly a result of post treatment modifications, which give a particular shift in pI and molecular weight. In addition, despite using cocktail protease inhibitors and DTT, protein cleavage or aggregation can happen. Table 1 contains a list of the protein names, encoding genes, UniProt base accession numbers, and Rt values. With regard to the Rts for the group means of relative spot volumes, the volume of a given spot in the control group was used as the denominator of the Rt parameter (Rt > 1.5, overexpression; Rt < 0.67, suppression). According to the results obtained with the Delta2D program, 8 of the 11 proteins were assigned to downregulated, and 3 of the 11 proteins were upregulated (Figure 1; Table 2). Figure 2 shows a fused image of 2DE gels with differentially expressed proteins in the AMD group versus the control group.

Table 1. Significantly ($p \leq 0.05$) differentially expressed proteins in neovascular age-related macular degeneration (AMD) patients as identified by MALDI-TOF MS. Listed molecular weights and pI values correspond to the MASCOT search results; carbamidomethylation of cysteine was a global modification. Rt (Ratio) quotient of the group means of relative spot volumes; volume of a given spot in control group is the denominator of the ratio parameter.

ID	Protein	Accession Number (UniProtKB)	Species	Score	Match	MW (Da)	pI	Seq. Cov (%)	Rt	p-Value
1	ATP-dependent translocase ABCB1	P08183	H. sapiens	87	11	141,788	9.06	9	2.193	0.025
5	Annexin A1	P04083	H. sapiens	96	12	38,918	6.57	41	0.664	0.026
6	Annexin A1	P04083	H. sapiens	59	9	38,918	6.57	30	0.575	0.017
8	Aldo-keto reductase family 1 member A1	P14550	H. sapiens	146	15	36,892	6.32	48	0.638	0.029
10	Retinal dehydrogenase 1	P00352	H. sapiens	75	9	55,454	6.30	24	2.027	0.011
12	Uncharacterized protein C11orf98	E9PRG8	H. sapiens	76	5	14,225	11.53	38	0.560	0.008
15	Glutathione S-transferase P	P09211	H. sapiens	89	8	23,569	5.43	50	0.529	0.007
23	Retinal dehydrogenase 1	P00352	H. sapiens	121	14	55,454	6.30	41	1.991	0.015
24	Alpha-enolase	P06733	H. sapiens	67	11	47,481	7.01	29	1.476	0.022
11	Annexin A4	P09525	H. sapiens	94	14	36,088	5.84	14	0.393	0.003
21	Annexin A1	P04083	H. sapiens	76	11	38,918	6.57	35	0.213	0.008
31	Allograft inflammatory factor 1	P55008	H. sapiens	77	5	16,693	5.97	34	0.560	0.026
33	Cytospin-A or Elongation factor 2	Q69YQ0 P13639	H. sapiens	113 88	16 12	124,925 96,246	5.52 6.41	16 12	0.560	0.037
32	Short stature homeobox protein 2	O60902	H. sapiens	65	5	35,160	8.99	12	0.529	0.041

Abbreviations: MW—molecular weight; pI—isoelectric point; Seq. Cov—sequence coverage; Rt—ratio.

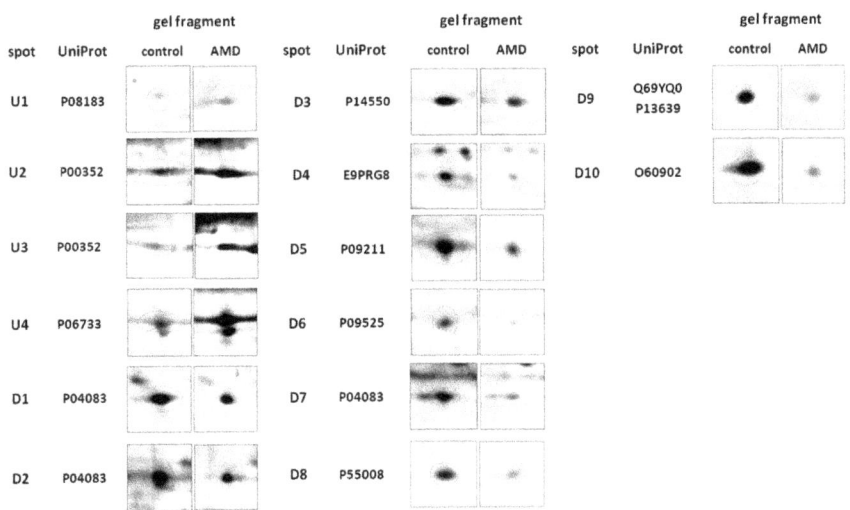

Figure 1. Representative 2DE gel spots of significantly ($p \leq 0.05$) differentially expressed proteins in Table 2. D software (version 4.7, DECODON, Greifswald, Germany). Left column represents the control group, and the right column represents the AMD group.

Table 2. AMD group up- and downregulated proteins.

Identified Protein	Upregulation or Downregulation	Fold Relative to Healthy Controls	Standard Deviation (SD)
Retinal dehydrogenase 1	Up	2.072 1.991	0.011 0.015
ATP-dependent translocase ABCB1	Up	2.193	0.025
Alpha-enolase	Up	1.476	0.022
Annexin A1	Down	0.664 0.575 0.213	0.026 0.017 0.008
Annexin A4	Down	0.393	0.003
Aldo-keto reductase family 1 member A1	Down	0.638	0.029
Uncharacterized protein C11orf98	Down	0.560	0.008
Glutathione S-transferase P	Down	0.529	0.007
Allograft inflammatory factor 1	Down	0.560	0.026
Cytospin-A or Elongation factor 2	Down	0.560	0.037
Short stature homeobox protein 2	Down	0.529	0.041

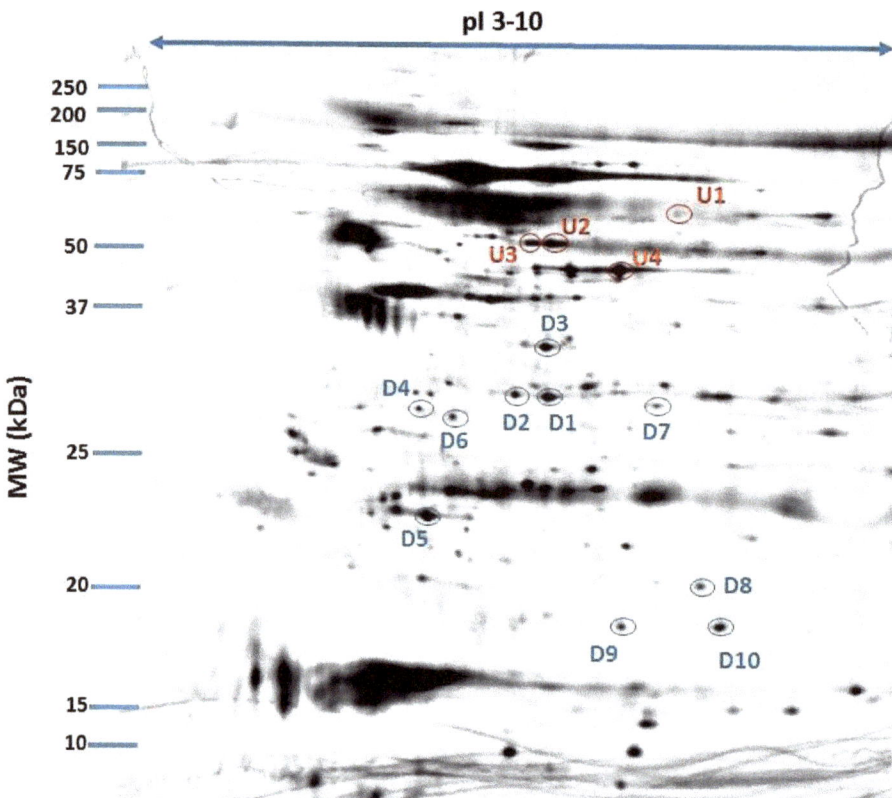

Figure 2. Fused image showing the condensed spot patterns from the experiment. The differentially expressed proteins in the neovascular AMD group versus the control group are marked. Upregulated proteins are indicated in red, and downregulated proteins are indicated in blue. The proteins were separated in the first dimension by isoelectric focusing over an isoelectric point (pI) range of 3–10. The second dimension was performed using 12.5% SDS polyacrylamide gels. The gels were silver stained, digitized, and processed in Delta2D software (version 4.7, DECODON).

4. Discussion

Currently, AMD is viewed as a disease involving impairment of multiple cellular processes; its exact pathogenesis remains unclear. Here, we found that proteins isolated from the tears of neovascular AMD patients were associated with oxidative stress, proteostasis regulation, inflammation, and neovascularization.

In our previous study [8], we identified 342 proteins that were differentially expressed in both types of AMD—atrophic and neovascular. We were, at that point in time, unable to perform a quantitative analysis of the obtained data. In the current manuscript, we quantified the identified proteins. This made it possible to pinpoint the proteins that could be more relevant for the disease progress. We also obtained a larger and more homogenous group—all of our patients presented an active stage of neovascular AMD.

4.1. Oxidative Stress

Oxidative stress (OS) occurs when there is an imbalance between reactive oxygen forms and the ability of a cell to neutralize their damaging effects through redox reactions. As a result, free radicals and superoxides damage cellular components and are especially harmful to proteins, lipids, and DNA. In healthy individuals, the retina has the greatest oxygen consumption per weight of any organ in the body, making it naturally vulnerable to OS [3,31,32]. In our study, we identified a number of proteins involved in OS induction and management in tear samples isolated from neovascular AMD patients. One of the most striking findings was the downregulation of glutathione S-transferase P. Glutathione (GSH) is one of the most important, ubiquitous antioxidant agents, whose role in the retinal anti-OS defense is well-established. It works by scavenging the reactive oxygen species and is a cofactor for GSH S-transferase P [9,10]. Its lowered concentration in the tear film of AMD patients may suggest the impaired cell-detoxification mechanisms.

Aldo-keto reductase family 1 member A1 (AKR1A1) is yet another protein involved in the cellular protection against OS, which was downregulated in our study, but its connection with the retina remains unclear [11,12].

Additionally, the identified protein retinal dehydrogenase 1 (RALDH1) is involved in redox reactions. Its key function is to oxidize retinaldehyde into retinoic acid, which participates in cell growth and differentiation and plays a critical role in the visual cycle [13].

Overall, the findings suggest that selected OS biomarkers can be found in tears from neovascular AMD patients.

4.2. Protein Clearance

Increased OS can damage proteins, and damaged proteins must be removed to prevent intracellular protein aggregation. Protein clearance impairment plays a crucial role in AMD development. Under normal conditions, retinal cells maintain proteostasis through two major mechanisms: proteasome-mediated degradation and lysosome-mediated autophagy. In AMD, impairment of phagocytosis leads to failure of the degradation of photoreceptor outer segments (POSs) in lysosomes, while impairment of autophagy leads to the accumulation of toxic protein aggregates and organelles, such as mitochondria [14]. Since RPE cells are quiescent cells, the consequences of deficient proteostasis are potentially devastating [15].

Annexin A1 and A4 are a part of the calcium-dependent phospholipid-binding family. Annexins A, beside regulating the inflammatory process described above, are vitally important to the autophagy process, and take an important part in the formation of the cytoskeleton, cell membrane, and in the cell signaling [16]. Annexin A1 is involved in the autophagosome-lysosome fusion, and its upregulation seems to inhibit autophagy process via PI3K/AKT activation followed by Beclin-1 and ATG5-dependent autophagy inhibition [17,18]. This may lead to the pathological aggregation of debris material within the RPE-BM complex, called drusen, and further stimuli for the formation of the choroidal neovascularization (CNV).

Given all of the above findings, the upregulation of the Annexin A1 and A4 in the tears of patients with neovascular AMD may indicate that proteostasis is disturbed in AMD.

4.3. Chronic Inflammation and Neovascularization

Increased inflammation is well established to occur during AMD pathogenesis in response to chronic OS and disturbed proteostasis [14]. Short lasting inflammation is a beneficial host defense in cells, while prolonged inflammation of low intensity (parainflammation) can lead to CNV and cell death in the context of AMD [19,20].

Annexin A1 (ANXA1) was found in our study on three different electrophoretic spots, probably to its further post treatment modification, which suggests its strong presence in the AMD tear film. Its concentration in the samples obtained from AMD patients was almost 5 times higher than in the control group. Previous studies investigating the ANXA1 impact on inflammation proved its significant anti-inflammatory potential [21–23]. It was also already found in the aqueous humor of the wet AMD patients (both Annexin A1 and A4) [24], in the drusen from the donors retina [25]. The impairment of the Annexins family function is related to numerous diseases, also neurodegenerative disorders and glaucoma, although in none it seems to be a primary cause [26–28].

Alpha-Enolase, which was found to be upregulated in our AMD patients' group, is another protein that can act as an autoantigen in the autoimmune process, which was already connected with AMD. Elevated levels of the antibodies against α-enolase were found in AMD patients' serum [29,30]. It is also strongly connected with the development of cancer-associated retinopathy (CAR), Alzheimer's disease (AD), cancer, and other diseases [31–33].

Another protein directly involved in inflammation and neovascularization process is allograft inflammatory factor 1 (AIF-1). In mouse models of neovascular AMD, it was highly expressed in an induced laser scarring spot, leading to NF-κB activation, and further CNV development [34]. It is also an established biomarker in local immune and inflammatory response of the retinal cells [35–37]. The questionable aspect is the downregulation of AIF-1 observed in our study, one would expect it to be upregulated.

Another hallmark of AMD is choroidal neovascularization (CNV), in which vessels sprout from the choroid and pass through the BM and the RPE, causing subretinal leakage, macular edema, and hemorrhages. In the end stage, a disciform scar is formed, with mesenchymal transition of RPE cells and general retinal disorganization. One of the key modulators of this process is VEGF, and the treatment of choice is anti-VEGF delivered via intravitreal injections. Although anti-VEGF administration has been a major breakthrough in AMD treatment, it has significant limitations: continued visits are necessary, macular scarring can occur, and patients can be refractory to treatment [38]. One of the proteins crucial for the BRB development, ATP-dependent translocase ABCB1, was found to be upregulated in our study. ABCB1 is responsible for the cellular transport, being an efflux pump, and is commonly associated with various types of cancers, due to its role in the multidrug resistance (MDR) [39–41].

Scarring is the eventual effect of the CNV presence, whether due to the treatment or the natural course of the disease. Elongation factor 2 was found to be downregulated in our AMD group. This protein was also identified in the Müller glia in course of the proliferative vitreoretinopathy, which is essentially a scarring process [42]. Elongation factors were also found to be downregulated in older retinas, which can partially explain its downregulation in our study [43].

Last of the identified proteins, short stature homeobox 2 has not been yet described in the context of AMD, or retinal dysfunction, and it should probably be concerned as an accidental finding. It was recently found that it may serve as a biomarker for bronchial squamous cell carcinoma (SCC) [44].

All these findings suggest a strong inflammatory component that can be observed in the tear film of AMD patients, which stays in line with our current knowledge of the disease.

4.4. Anti-VEGF Treatment

All of the patients included in our study were treated with intraocular anti-VEGF injections over the course of a national drug program. This warranted quality patient selection and confirmation of medical history. The patients were first qualified by a local ophthalmologist, and then the diagnosis was confirmed online by nationally board-certified retinal AMD specialists. In all cases, the samples were collected at the follow-up day before the anti-VEGF injection. Therefore, each patient was examined 28 to 31 days after previous anti-VEGF treatment. Since we did not include treatment-naïve patients with AMD, anti-VEGF treatment might have affected the protein expression results. This may explain why we did not observe differential expression of certain proteins, such as VEGF or PDGF, even though differences in such proteins have been found in other studies [45,46]. On the other hand, this might have enabled the roles and differential expression of other proteins involved in neovascularization. The VEGF pathway, although extremely important, is certainly not the sole promotor of the growth of the new vessels. Preferably, a larger clinical study should be conducted on samples collected from patients at different stages of AMD progression.

4.5. Limitations of the Study

One major limitation of our study is the correlation between the tear film composition and macular lesions. Although the tear film is not directly connected with the retina, it can be altered by the partial blood–retinal barrier breakdown (BRB) in the course of AMD. BRB was mainly described in diabetic retinopathy, and functions as a key factor in this disease, but the BRB can also be found in the neovascular AMD, where macular edema, subretinal fluid, and vitreous hemorrhages are present [47–50]. Thus, we believe that in an active phase of neovascular AMD, it is possible that the leakage from the pathological vessels can be also detected in the tear film.

Another limitation of this study is that being a pilot study, we were not able to analyze enough samples to reach adequate power of the tests used in statistical calculations. According to an amount of wet AMD cases in our region, we would need over 300 samples for each group. This will be done in the following experiments.

5. Conclusions

Tear film is a well-established material for obtaining biomarkers of various diseases. We believe that the findings of this study enhance the current understanding of AMD as a multifactorial disease with underlying persistent OS, cell clearance mechanism impairment, inflammation, and CNV. Although the identified proteins probably should not be considered verified biomarkers, the differences in their expression between groups suggest that they are connected to ongoing pathological processes in the macula and tear film. Further studies are needed to confirm this possibility, preferably studies comparing the levels of specific proteins in different body fluids, such as the plasma, aqueous humor, and tear film.

Supplementary Materials: Supplementary materials can be found at https://www.mdpi.com/article/10.3390/jcm10143060/s1. Supplementary Table S1: Characteristics of wet AMD patients. Supplementary, Table S2: Characteristics of control group patients.

Author Contributions: Conceptualization, M.W.; methodology, M.W., K.M., and S.W.; software, K.M.; validation, M.W., K.M., and Ł.A.; formal analysis, M.W.; investigation, M.W.; resources, M.W., D.W., and S.W.; data curation, M.W.; writing—original draft preparation, M.W.; writing—review and editing, M.W., K.K., D.W., and S.W.; visualization, K.M.; supervision, K.K. and J.M.; project administration, M.W.; funding acquisition, M.W. All authors have read and agreed to the published version of the manuscript.

Funding: This work was supported by the Polish National Science Centre (NCN). M.W. was supported by Preludium grant number UMO-2017/25/N/NZ5/01875. D.W. was supported by Preludium grant number UMO-2016/23/N/NZ5/02576. The research materials supporting this publication can be accessed by contacting the corresponding authors.

Institutional Review Board Statement: Ethical review and approval were waived for this study, due to the standard procedure of tear film collection and non-invasive nature of the experiment.

Informed Consent Statement: Informed consent was obtained from all subjects involved in the study.

Data Availability Statement: Data available after contacting corresponding author: mateuszwiniarczyk@umlub.pl.

Conflicts of Interest: The authors declare no conflict of interest.

References

1. Li, K.; Chen, Z.; Duan, F.; Liang, J.; Wu, K. Quantification of Tear Proteins by SDS-PAGE with an Internal Standard Protein: A New Method with Special Reference to Small Volume Tears. *Graefes Arch. Clin. Exp. Ophthalmol.* **2010**, *248*, 853–862. [CrossRef] [PubMed]
2. Posa, A.; Bräuer, L.; Schicht, M.; Garreis, F.; Beileke, S.; Paulsen, F. Schirmer Strip vs. Capillary Tube Method: Non-Invasive Methods of Obtaining Proteins from Tear Fluid. *Ann. Anat.* **2013**, *195*, 137–142. [CrossRef] [PubMed]
3. Green-Church, K.B.; Nichols, K.K.; Kleinholz, N.M.; Zhang, L.; Nichols, J.J. Investigation of the Human Tear Film Proteome Using Multiple Proteomic Approaches. *Mol. Vis.* **2008**, *14*, 456–470.

4. González, N.; Iloro, I.; Durán, J.A.; Elortza, F.; Suárez, T. Evaluation of Inter-Day and Inter-Individual Variability of Tear Peptide/Protein Profiles by MALDI-TOF MS Analyses. *Mol. Vis.* **2012**, *18*, 1572–1582.
5. Rentka, A.; Koroskenyi, K.; Harsfalvi, J.; Szekanecz, Z.; Szucs, G.; Szodoray, P.; Kemeny-Beke, A. Evaluation of Commonly Used Tear Sampling Methods and Their Relevance in Subsequent Biochemical Analysis. *Ann. Clin. Biochem.* **2017**, *54*, 521–529. [CrossRef]
6. Ablamowicz, A.F.; Nichols, J.J. Concentrations of MUC16 and MUC5AC Using Three Tear Collection Methods. *Mol. Vis.* **2017**, *23*, 529–537.
7. Shevchenko, A.; Wilm, M.; Vorm, O.; Mann, M. Mass Spectrometric Sequencing of Proteins Silver-Stained Polyacrylamide Gels. *Anal. Chem.* **1996**, *68*, 850–858. [CrossRef]
8. Winiarczyk, M.; Kaarniranta, K.; Winiarczyk, S.; Adaszek, Ł.; Winiarczyk, D.; Mackiewicz, J. Tear Film Proteome in Age-Related Macular Degeneration. *Graefe's Arch. Clin. Exp. Ophthalmol.* **2018**, *256*, 1127–1139. [CrossRef] [PubMed]
9. Tew, K.D. Redox in Redux: Emergent Roles for Glutathione S-Transferase P (GSTP) in Regulation of Cell Signaling and S-Glutathionylation. *Biochem. Pharmacol.* **2007**, *73*, 1257–1269. [CrossRef] [PubMed]
10. Sreekumar, P.G.; Ferrington, D.A.; Kannan, R. Glutathione Metabolism and the Novel Role of Mitochondrial GSH in Retinal Degeneration. *Antioxidants* **2021**, *10*, 661. [CrossRef]
11. Chen, W.-R.; Lan, Y.-W.; Chen, H.-L.; Chen, C.-M. AKR1A1 Deficiency Is Associated with High Risk of Alcohol-Induced Fatty Liver Syndrome. *FASEB J.* **2018**, *32*, 546.6. [CrossRef]
12. Stomberski, C.T.; Anand, P.; Venetos, N.M.; Hausladen, A.; Zhou, H.-L.; Premont, R.T.; Stamler, J.S. AKR1A1 Is a Novel Mammalian S-Nitroso-Glutathione Reductase. *J. Biol. Chem.* **2019**, *294*, 18285–18293. [CrossRef]
13. Morgan, C.A.; Hurley, T.D. Characterization of Two Distinct Structural Classes of Selective Aldehyde Dehydrogenase 1A1 Inhibitors. *J. Med. Chem.* **2015**, *58*, 1964–1975. [CrossRef]
14. Kaarniranta, K.; Uusitalo, H.; Blasiak, J.; Felszeghy, S.; Kannan, R.; Kauppinen, A.; Salminen, A.; Sinha, D.; Ferrington, D. Mechanisms of Mitochondrial Dysfunction and Their Impact on Age-Related Macular Degeneration. *Progress Retin. Eye Res.* **2020**, *100858*. [CrossRef]
15. Ferrington, D.A.; Sinha, D.; Kaarniranta, K. Defects in Retinal Pigment Epithelial Cell Proteolysis and the Pathology Associated with Age-Related Macular Degeneration. *Progress Retin. Eye Res.* **2016**, *51*, 69–89. [CrossRef] [PubMed]
16. Xi, Y.; Ju, R.; Wang, Y. Roles of Annexin A Protein Family in Autophagy Regulation and Therapy. *Biomed. Pharmacother.* **2020**, *130*, 110591. [CrossRef] [PubMed]
17. Zhu, J.-F.; Huang, W.; Yi, H.-M.; Xiao, T.; Li, J.-Y.; Feng, J.; Yi, H.; Lu, S.-S.; Li, X.-H.; Lu, R.-H.; et al. Annexin A1-Suppressed Autophagy Promotes Nasopharyngeal Carcinoma Cell Invasion and Metastasis by PI3K/AKT Signaling Activation. *Cell Death Dis.* **2018**, *9*, 1–16. [CrossRef] [PubMed]
18. White, I.J.; Bailey, L.M.; Aghakhani, M.R.; Moss, S.E.; Futter, C.E. EGF Stimulates Annexin 1-Dependent Inward Vesiculation in a Multivesicular Endosome Subpopulation. *EMBO J.* **2006**, *25*, 1–12. [CrossRef]
19. Datta, S.; Cano, M.; Ebrahimi, K.; Wang, L.; Handa, J.T. The Impact of Oxidative Stress and Inflammation on RPE Degeneration in Non-Neovascular AMD. *Progress Retin. Eye Res.* **2017**, *60*, 201–218. [CrossRef]
20. Kauppinen, A.; Paterno, J.J.; Blasiak, J.; Salminen, A.; Kaarniranta, K. Inflammation and Its Role in Age-Related Macular Degeneration. *Cell Mol. Life Sci.* **2016**, *73*, 1765–1786. [CrossRef]
21. D'Acquisto, F.; Merghani, A.; Lecona, E.; Rosignoli, G.; Raza, K.; Buckley, C.D.; Flower, R.J.; Perretti, M. Annexin-1 Modulates T-Cell Activation and Differentiation. *Blood* **2007**, *109*, 1095–1102. [CrossRef]
22. Sanches, J.M.; Correia-Silva, R.D.; Duarte, G.H.B.; Fernandes, A.M.A.P.; Sánchez-Vinces, S.; Carvalho, P.O.; Oliani, S.M.; Bortoluci, K.R.; Moreira, V.; Gil, C.D. Role of Annexin A1 in NLRP3 Inflammasome Activation in Murine Neutrophils. *Cells* **2021**, *10*, 121. [CrossRef] [PubMed]
23. Yazid, S.; Gardner, P.J.; Carvalho, L.; Chu, C.J.; Flower, R.J.; Solito, E.; Lee, R.W.J.; Ali, R.R.; Dick, A.D. Annexin-A1 Restricts Th17 Cells and Attenuates the Severity of Autoimmune Disease. *J. Autoimmun.* **2015**, *58*, 1–11. [CrossRef] [PubMed]
24. Kang, G.-Y.; Bang, J.Y.; Choi, A.J.; Yoon, J.; Lee, W.-C.; Choi, S.; Yoon, S.; Kim, H.C.; Baek, J.-H.; Park, H.S.; et al. Exosomal Proteins in the Aqueous Humor as Novel Biomarkers in Patients with Neovascular Age-Related Macular Degeneration. *J. Proteome Res.* **2014**, *13*, 581–595. [CrossRef] [PubMed]
25. Crabb, J.W.; Miyagi, M.; Gu, X.; Shadrach, K.; West, K.A.; Sakaguchi, H.; Kamei, M.; Hasan, A.; Yan, L.; Rayborn, M.E.; et al. Drusen Proteome Analysis: An Approach to the Etiology of Age-Related Macular Degeneration. *Proc. Natl. Acad. Sci. USA* **2002**, *99*, 14682–14687. [CrossRef]
26. Yang, Z.; Quigley, H.A.; Pease, M.E.; Yang, Y.; Qian, J.; Valenta, D.; Zack, D.J. Changes in Gene Expression in Experimental Glaucoma and Optic Nerve Transection: The Equilibrium between Protective and Detrimental Mechanisms. *Investig. Ophthalmol. Vis. Sci.* **2007**, *48*, 5539–5548. [CrossRef] [PubMed]
27. Iaccarino, L.; Ghirardello, A.; Canova, M.; Zen, M.; Bettio, S.; Nalotto, L.; Punzi, L.; Doria, A. Anti-Annexins Autoantibodies: Their Role as Biomarkers of Autoimmune Diseases. *Autoimmun. Rev.* **2011**, *10*, 553–558. [CrossRef]
28. Cañas, F.; Simonin, L.; Couturaud, F.; Renaudineau, Y. Annexin A2 Autoantibodies in Thrombosis and Autoimmune Diseases. *Thromb. Res.* **2015**, *135*, 226–230. [CrossRef]
29. Adamus, G.; Chew, E.Y.; Ferris, F.L.; Klein, M.L. Prevalence of Anti-Retinal Autoantibodies in Different Stages of Age-Related Macular Degeneration. *BMC Ophthalmol.* **2014**, *14*, 154. [CrossRef]

30. Joachim, S.C.; Bruns, K.; Lackner, K.J.; Pfeiffer, N.; Grus, F.H. Analysis of IgG Antibody Patterns against Retinal Antigens and Antibodies to α-Crystallin, GFAP, and α-Enolase in Sera of Patients with "Wet" Age-Related Macular Degeneration. *Graefe's Arch. Clin. Exp. Ophthalmol.* **2006**, *245*, 619. [CrossRef]
31. Adamus, G.; Aptsiauri, N.; Guy, J.; Heckenlively, J.; Flannery, J.; Hargrave, P.A. The Occurrence of Serum Autoantibodies against Enolase in Cancer-Associated Retinopathy. *Clin. Immunol. Immunopathol.* **1996**, *78*, 120–129. [CrossRef]
32. Dot, C.; Guigay, J.; Adamus, G. Anti-α-Enolase Antibodies in Cancer-Associated Retinopathy with Small Cell Carcinoma of the Lung. *Am. J. Ophthalmol.* **2005**, *139*, 746–747. [CrossRef] [PubMed]
33. Morohoshi, K.; Goodwin, A.M.; Ohbayashi, M.; Ono, S.J. Autoimmunity in Retinal Degeneration: Autoimmune Retinopathy and Age-Related Macular Degeneration. *J. Autoimmun.* **2009**, *33*, 247–254. [CrossRef] [PubMed]
34. Hikage, F.; Lennikov, A.; Mukwaya, A.; Lachota, M.; Ida, Y.; Utheim, T.P.; Chen, D.F.; Huang, H.; Ohguro, H. NF-KB Activation in Retinal Microglia Is Involved in the Inflammatory and Neovascularization Signaling in Laser-Induced Choroidal Neovascularization in Mice. *Exp. Cell Res.* **2021**, *403*, 112581. [CrossRef] [PubMed]
35. Singh, R.K.; Occelli, L.M.; Binette, F.; Petersen-Jones, S.M.; Nasonkin, I.O. Transplantation of Human Embryonic Stem Cell-Derived Retinal Tissue in the Subretinal Space of the Cat Eye. *Stem Cells Dev.* **2019**, *28*, 1151–1166. [CrossRef] [PubMed]
36. Hambright, D.; Park, K.-Y.; Brooks, M.; McKay, R.; Swaroop, A.; Nasonkin, I.O. Long-Term Survival and Differentiation of Retinal Neurons Derived from Human Embryonic Stem Cell Lines in Un-Immunosuppressed Mouse Retina. *Mol. Vis.* **2012**, *18*, 920–936.
37. Stifter, J.; Ulbrich, F.; Goebel, U.; Böhringer, D.; Lagrèze, W.A.; Biermann, J. Neuroprotection and Neuroregeneration of Retinal Ganglion Cells after Intravitreal Carbon Monoxide Release. *PLoS ONE* **2017**, *12*, e0188444. [CrossRef] [PubMed]
38. Ambati, J.; Fowler, B.J. Mechanisms of Age-Related Macular Degeneration. *Neuron* **2012**, *75*, 26–39. [CrossRef]
39. Gutmann, D.A.P.; Ward, A.; Urbatsch, I.L.; Chang, G.; van Veen, H.W. Understanding Polyspecificity of Multidrug ABC Transporters: Closing in on the Gaps in ABCB1. *Trends Biochem. Sci.* **2010**, *35*, 36–42. [CrossRef]
40. Hodges, L.M.; Markova, S.M.; Chinn, L.W.; Gow, J.M.; Kroetz, D.L.; Klein, T.E.; Altman, R.B. Very Important Pharmacogene Summary: ABCB1 (MDR1, P-Glycoprotein). *Pharmacogenet Genom.* **2011**, *21*, 152–161. [CrossRef]
41. Lee, W.-K.; Frank, T. Teaching an Old Dog New Tricks: Reactivated Developmental Signaling Pathways Regulate ABCB1 and Chemoresistance in Cancer. *Cancer Drug Resist.* **2021**, *4*. [CrossRef]
42. Eastlake, K.; Heywood, W.E.; Banerjee, P.; Bliss, E.; Mills, K.; Khaw, P.T.; Charteris, D.; Limb, G.A. Comparative Proteomic Analysis of Normal and Gliotic PVR Retina and Contribution of Müller Glia to This Profile. *Exp. Eye Res.* **2018**, *177*, 197–207. [CrossRef]
43. Mirzaei, M.; Pushpitha, K.; Deng, L.; Chitranshi, N.; Gupta, V.; Rajput, R.; Mangani, A.B.; Dheer, Y.; Godinez, A.; McKay, M.J.; et al. Upregulation of Proteolytic Pathways and Altered Protein Biosynthesis Underlie Retinal Pathology in a Mouse Model of Alzheimer's Disease. *Mol. Neurobiol.* **2019**, *56*, 6017–6034. [CrossRef] [PubMed]
44. Ni, S.; Ye, M.; Huang, T. Short Stature Homeobox 2 Methylation as a Potential Noninvasive Biomarker in Bronchial Aspirates for Lung Cancer Diagnosis. *Oncotarget* **2017**, *8*, 61253–61263. [CrossRef] [PubMed]
45. Ang, W.J.; Zunaina, E.; Norfadzillah, A.J.; Raja-Norliza, R.O.; Julieana, M.; Ab-Hamid, S.A.; Mahaneem, M. Evaluation of Vascular Endothelial Growth Factor Levels in Tears and Serum among Diabetic Patients. *PLoS ONE* **2019**, *14*. [CrossRef] [PubMed]
46. Rentka, A.; Hársfalvi, J.; Berta, A.; Köröskényi, K.; Szekanecz, Z.; Szűcs, G.; Szodoray, P.; Kemény-Beke, Á. Vascular Endothelial Growth Factor in Tear Samples of Patients with Systemic Sclerosis. *Mediators Inflamm.* **2015**, *2015*. [CrossRef] [PubMed]
47. Klaassen, I.; Van Noorden, C.J.F.; Schlingemann, R.O. Molecular Basis of the Inner Blood-Retinal Barrier and Its Breakdown in Diabetic Macular Edema and Other Pathological Conditions. *Progress Retin. Eye Res.* **2013**, *34*, 19–48. [CrossRef] [PubMed]
48. Schlingemann, R.O. Role of Growth Factors and the Wound Healing Response in Age-Related Macular Degeneration. *Graefes Arch. Clin. Exp. Ophthalmol.* **2004**, *242*, 91–101. [CrossRef]
49. El-Mollayess, G.M.; Noureddine, B.N.; Bashshur, Z.F. Bevacizumab and Neovascular Age Related Macular Degeneration: Pathogenesis and Treatment. *Semin. Ophthalmol.* **2011**, *26*, 69–76. [CrossRef]
50. Gawęcki, M.; Jaszczuk-Maciejewska, A.; Jurska-Jaśko, A.; Kneba, M.; Grzybowski, A. Transfoveal Micropulse Laser Treatment of Central Serous Chorioretinopathy within Six Months of Disease Onset. *J. Clin. Med.* **2019**, *8*, 1398. [CrossRef]

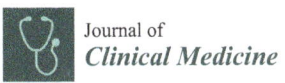

Article

Clinical Outcome and Drug Expenses of Intravitreal Therapy for Diabetic Macular Edema: A Retrospective Study in Sardinia, Italy

Chiara Altana [1], Matthew Gavino Donadu [1,2,*], Stefano Dore [3,4], Giacomo Boscia [4], Gabriella Carmelita [1], Stefania Zanetti [2], Francesco Boscia [5] and Antonio Pinna [3,4]

1. Hospital Pharmacy, Azienda Ospedaliero Universitaria di Sassari, 07100 Sassari, Italy; chiara.altana@aousassari.it (C.A.); gabriella.carmelita@aousassari.it (G.C.)
2. Department of Biomedical Sciences, University of Sassari, 07100 Sassari, Italy; zanettis@uniss.it
3. Ophthalmology Unit, Azienda Ospedaliero Universitaria di Sassari, 07100 Sassari, Italy; stefanodore@hotmail.com (S.D.); apinna@uniss.it (A.P.)
4. Department of Medical, Surgical and Experimental Sciences, University of Sassari, 07100 Sassari, Italy; bosciagiacomo@gmail.com
5. Section of Ophthalmology, Department of Basic Medical Science, Neuroscience and Sense Organs, University of Bari, 70124 Bari, Italy; francescoboscia@hotmail.com
* Correspondence: mdonadu@uniss.it

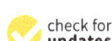

Abstract: Background: Diabetic macular edema (DME) is a leading cause of visual loss in working-age adults. The purpose of this retrospective study was to perform an epidemiological analysis on DME patients treated with intravitreal drugs in a tertiary hospital. The clinical outcome, adverse drug reactions (ADRs), and intravitreal drug expenses were assessed. Methods: All DME patients treated with Ranibizumab, Aflibercept, Dexamethasone implant, and Fluocinolone Acetonide implant at the Sassari University Hospital, Italy, between January 2017 and June 2020 were included. Central macular thickness (CMT) and best corrected visual acuity (BCVA) were measured. ADRs and drug expenses were analyzed. Results: Two-hundred thirty-one DME patients (mean age: 65 years) received intravitreal agents. Mean CMT and BCVA were 380 µm and 0.5 LogMAR at baseline, 298 µm and 0.44 logMAR after one year ($p = 0.04$), and 295 µm and 0.4 logMAR at the end of the follow-up period. A total of 1501 intravitreal injections were given; no major ADRs were reported. Treatment cost was €915,000 (€261,429/year). Twenty non-responders to Ranibizumab or Aflibercept were switched to a Dexamethasone implant. In these patients, mean CMT and BCVA were 468 µm and 0.5 LogMar at the time of switching and 362 µm and 0.3 LogMar at the end of the follow-up ($p = 0.00014$ and $p = 0.08$, respectively). Conclusion: Results confirm that Ranibizumab, Aflibercept, and Dexamethasone implant are effective and safe in DME treatment. A switch to Dexamethasone implant for patients receiving Aflibercept or Ranibizumab with minimal/no clinical benefit should be considered.

Keywords: diabetic macular edema; intravitreal agents; best corrected visual acuity; central retinal thickness; adverse drug reactions; intravitreal drug expenses

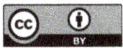

1. Introduction

Diabetic macular edema (DME) is one of the most severe complications of diabetic retinopathy and the main reason for legal blindness among working-age individuals in developed countries [1,2].

Population-based studies have reported DME prevalence rates of 4.2% to 7.9% in type 1 diabetic patients and 1.4% to 12.8% in type 2 diabetic patients [3]. In a Cochrane review of the DME prevalence evaluated using optical coherence tomography (OCT), the prevalence rates covered a wider range (19–65%) [4].

Worldwide, the prevalence rate for diabetic retinopathy has been estimated at 34.6% (93 million people) [5]. In the U.S., the prevalence rate for retinopathy for all diabetic patients aged ≥40 years has been reported to be 28.5% (4.2 million people) [5]. The prevalence of diabetic retinopathy increases with increasing duration of disease [6].

In the Wisconsin Epidemiologic Study of Diabetic Retinopathy, the four-year incidence of diabetic retinopathy was 59% when age at diagnosis was <30 years [7]. Conversely, when age at diagnosis was ≥30 years, the incidence rate was 47% in insulin users and 34% in nonusers of insulin [8].

In diabetic retinopathy, structural changes of the retinal vascular network can be observed, leading to accumulation of fluids in the macular region, disruption of the blood-retinal barrier, and expression of various inflammatory factors, including the vascular endothelial growth factor (VEGF), intercellular adhesion molecules (ICAM-1), monocyte chemoattractant protein (MCP-1), interleukine-6, and others [9,10]. Recently, experimental and clinical evidence have shown that in addition to microvascular changes and inflammation, retinal neurodegeneration may contribute to retinal damage in the early stages of diabetic retinopathy [11]. In the most advanced stages, a proliferative diabetic retinopathy can occur, which may result in a vitreous hemorrhage and/or tractional retinal detachment [12,13].

In patients with DME, anti-VEGF agents and corticosteroids are the gold standard of therapy. The purpose of this study was to carry out an epidemiological analysis on DME patients treated with intravitreal drugs (anti-VEGF agents and corticosteroid-based implants) between January 2017 and June 2020 at the Sassari University Hospital, Northwest Sardinia, Italy. Specifically, the clinical outcome, therapy adherence, and drug expenses were assessed.

2. Materials and Methods

2.1. Participants

All 231 DME patients (139 men, 92 women; mean age: 65 years) treated with intravitreal drugs at the Ophthalmology Unit—Azienda Ospedaliero-Universitaria, Sassari, Italy, between January 2017 and June 2020 were included in this retrospective study.

Our unit has a catchment population of approximately 335,000 living in an area of 4300 square kilometers (Sassari province).

Ethical approval was waived by the local Ethics Committee of the Azienda Ospedaliero-Universitaria di Sassari in view of the retrospective nature of the survey, which was conducted in full accord with the tenets of the Declaration of Helsinki. Each participant received detailed information and provided informed consent.

Affected eyes received a loading dose of three consecutive monthly intravitreal injections of Ranumizumab (0.3 mg) or five consecutive monthly injections of Aflibercept (2.0 mg), followed by a treat-and-extend regimen. This regimen incorporates elements of both monthly and as-needed (PRN) treatment regimens. As with a monthly regimen, the ophthalmologist administers anti-VEGF intravitreal injections at each follow-up examination, but instead of a fixed 4-week follow-up interval, the length of the interval varies according to disease activity.

In patients presenting a serous detachment of neuroepithelium and/or a poor response in terms of improvement of best corrected visual acuity (BCVA) and central macular thickness (CMT) three months after the loading phase with Ranimizumab or Aflibercept, intravitreal therapy was switched to a Dexamethasone implant (700 μg), administered twice yearly, or to a Fluocinolone Acetonide implant (190 μg).

2.2. Data Analysis

Data regarding treatments were extracted from the Eye Clinic records, web-based monitoring records by the Italian Medicines Agency (Agenzia Italiana del Farmaco-AIFA), and data flows included in the New Health Information System (Nuovo Sistema Informativo Sanitario—NSIS).

Data about the treatment period (months) and regimen were extracted from AIFA web-based monitoring records. In addition, the analysis also yielded information regarding the number and types of therapy switches during the period under analysis. Furthermore, the study verified adherence of treatments to therapy protocols, assessing the number of injections performed.

Evaluation of treatment efficacy was based on the measurement of CMT expressed in μm and BCVA expressed in logMAR. CMT data were obtained by using Topcon OCT 2000 (Japan). The analysis compared clinical parameters at baseline, after the first year, and at the end of the follow-up period. Evaluation of data on efficacy was carried out only for patients who received at least one year of therapy.

Data on safety were evaluated as the number and severity of suspected adverse reactions to drugs (Adverse Drug Reactions, ADRs) observed during analysis of clinical documents.

Costs of intravitreal drugs under analysis were extracted by the IT System of the Sardinian Region adopted by all healthcare facilities in Sardinia.

For drugs not monitored by AIFA (corticosteroids), the epidemiological analysis was conducted on data obtained from the patients' clinical records.

2.3. Statistical Analysis

Qualitative data are shown as number and percentages. The analyzed data showed a normal distribution (Kolmogorov–Smirnov test); hence, the Student's t-test for continuous variables was used. A p-value < 0.05 was considered statistically significant. The analysis was carried out by using IBM SPSS Statistics 24 for Windows.

3. Results

The number of patients with bilateral DME was 78 (34%) out of 231. The total number of DME eyes treated with intravitreal drugs was 309. Each eye received on average 4.5 intravitreal injections per year. Overall, the total number of intravitreal injections administered for DME treatment during the period under analysis was 1501, with an average of 375 injections per year. The most used agent was Ranibizumab (46%), followed by Aflibercept (34%) and Dexamethasone implant (20%), while Fluocinolone Acetonide intravitreal implants accounted for less than 1% of administrations (Table 1). Dexamethasone and Fluocinolone Acetonide implants were never used as first line therapy.

Table 1. Intravitreal agents used in the treatment of diabetic macular edema (DME).

Drug	Average Number (%) of Intravitreal Injections per Year
Ranibizumab	172 (45.85%)
Aflibercept	127 (34%)
Dexamethasone implant	76 (20%)
Fluocinolone Acetonide implant	2 (0.15%)
Bevacizumab	0%

Adherence to therapy was evaluated as number of interruptions before the end of the loading phase (three doses with 4-week intervals for Ranibizumab and five doses with 4-week intervals for Aflibercept). The rate of interruptions was 12%, with 10% represented by Ranibizumab. During the analyzed period, a total of 34 therapy switches occurred. Ranibizumab or Aflibercept was switched to a Dexamethasone implant in 20 (59%) cases, whereas a switch to a Fluocinolone Acetonide implant was performed in two (6%).

The mean CMT at baseline was 380 μm. After the first year of therapy, the mean CMT was 298 μm, with an 82 μm reduction ($p = 0.04$). At the end of the follow-up period, the mean CMT remained substantially unchanged (295 μm). The mean BCVA was 0.5 LogMAR at baseline, 0.44 logMAR after one year of treatment ($p = 0.04$), and 0.4 logMAR at the end of treatment. CMT and BCVA values for all patients are summarized in Figure 1.

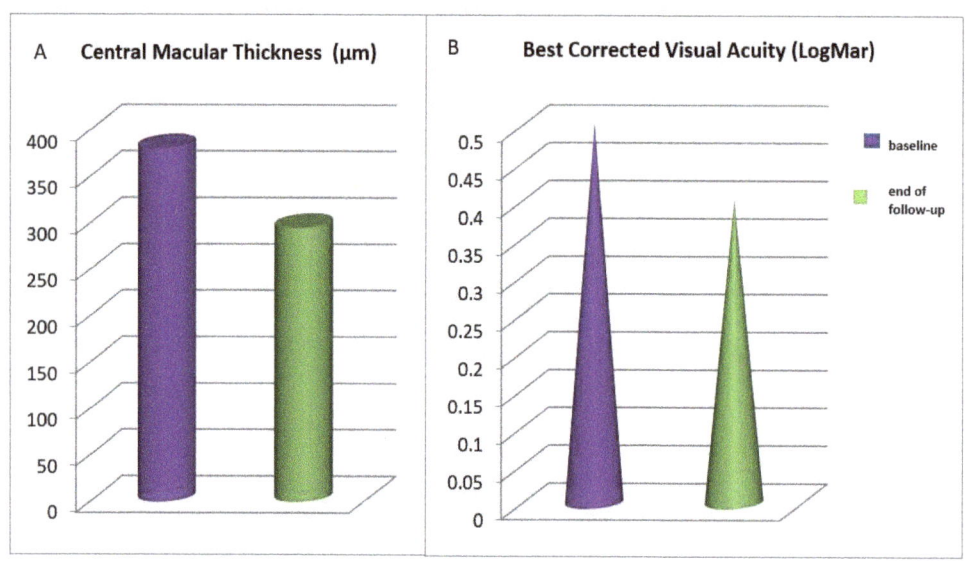

Figure 1. Central macular thickness (**A**) and best corrected visual acuity (**B**) values at baseline and at the end of the follow-up for all patients receiving intravitreal treatment for diabetic macular edema.

In the 20 patients switched to a Dexamethasone implant, the mean CMT was 468 μm at the time of switching and 362 μm at the end of the follow-up, a statistically significant difference ($p = 0.00014$). The mean BCVA was 0.5 LogMar at the time of switching and 0.3 LogMar at the end of the follow-up, again a statistically significant difference ($p = 0.08$). CMT and BCVA values before and after the switch to Dexamethasone are shown in Figure 2.

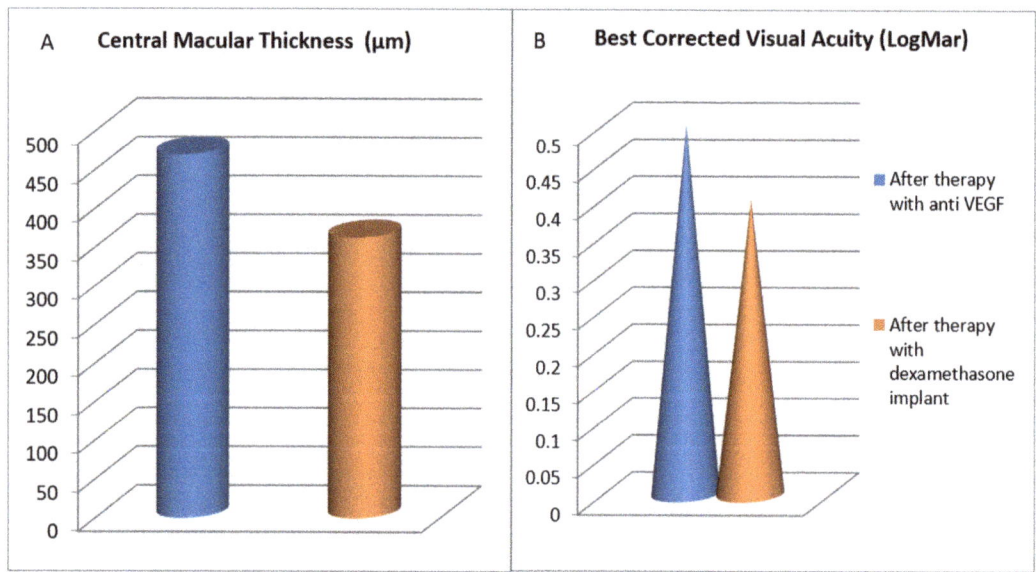

Figure 2. Central macular thickness (**A**) and best corrected visual acuity (**B**) values at the time of switching to a Dexamethasone implant and at the end of the follow-up.

Considering all types of retinal diseases for which intravitreal drugs are used (i.e., wet age-related macular degeneration, retinal vein occlusion, myopic choroidal neovascularization, etc.), the total treatment cost during the analyzed period amounted to €5,780,000 (Table 2), with an average cost of €1,651,429 per year. As far as DME is concerned, the global cost of intravitreal treatment was €915,000, with an average cost of €261,429 per year, accounting for approximately 16% of total expenses. It is important to emphasize that the total expense per year is subject to high variability, due to differences in drug consumption and selling price, with the latter decreasing over the years. Ranibizumab was the drug that mostly affected the expense, as it was the most prescribed intravitreal agent (46%), followed by Aflibercept (34%).

Table 2. Annual number and cost of intravitreal (IV) injections in the period January 2017–June 2020.

Year	All IV Injections (n.)	Global IV Cost (€)	IV Injections for DME	IV Cost for DME * (€)
2017	2416	1,180,000.00€	358	175,000.00€
2018	2720	1,750,000.00€	388	250,000.00€
2019	2642	1,600,000.00€	643	390,000.00€
2020 [†]	1395	1,250,000.00€	112	100,000.00€
TOTAL	9173	5,780,000.00€	1501	915,000.00€

* DME = Diabetic Macular Edema; [†] January–June.

Our study showed that the analyzed treatments were generally well tolerated. Indeed, during the period taken into consideration, no major ADRs (endophthalmitis, occlusive vasculitis, etc.) were reported.

4. Discussion

DME represents a social burden due to the reduction of vision and lower quality of life of patients affected [1,2]. Our retrospective survey confirms the clinical efficacy of Ranibizumab, Aflibercept, and Dexamethasone implant in the treatment of DME [5,14,15], with significant BCVA improvement and CRT reduction, especially after the first year of treatment. In terms of safety, the drugs analyzed showed a good risk-benefits outcome, with no systemic ADRs. Occasionally, local reactions were reported, mostly related to the injection procedure and not connected to pharmacologic properties of the intravitreal agents. It is important to emphasize that no thromboembolic events were observed during the analyzed period. On the other hand, data related to adherence to therapy showed that as much as 12% of the patients did not complete the loading phase, with a negative impact on the outcome. The greatest contribution to this value was given by Ranibizumab, the most used anti-VEGF agent in this investigation. Unfortunately, from the available data, it was not possible to ascertain the reason of treatment interruption in most cases.

In our study, 20 patients receiving intravitreal Ranimizumab or Aflibercept with disappointing results were switched to a Dexamethasone implant. After switching, there was a significant improvement in the mean BCVA (from 0.5 to 0.3 LogMar) and CMT (from 468 to 362 μm).

In patients presenting a serous detachment of neuroepithelium and poor response in terms of BCVA and CMT after the loading phase with Ranimizumab or Aflibercept, intravitreal injection of a Dexamethasone implant should be considered. This can be administered as an adjunctive treatment, without suspending the anti-VEGF agents, or as a switch treatment.

Overall, expenses for DME treatment accounted for only 16% of the global cost of all intravitreal injections for any cause. This can at least in part be explained by the fact that about one-third of diabetic patients are not aware of having the disease; therefore, diabetic retinopathy and DME are commonly underdiagnosed [5]. Cost analysis did not show a linear trend over time, presenting a peak in 2018. In 2020, the expenses were considerably lower, as eye examinations and intravitreal injections fell due to the hospital emergency created by the first COVID-19 wave; furthermore, there was a reduction in the selling price of all the intravitreal agents used.

Our study has important limitations, including its retrospective nature and the use of relatively crude estimates of hospital expenses. However, it provides some new data in an underinvestigated topic, such as the drug expenses of intravitreal treatment for DME.

5. Conclusions

In conclusion, our results confirm that Ranibizumab, Aflibercept, and Dexamethasone implant are effective and safe in the treatment of DME. A therapy switch to Dexamethasone implant for patients receiving Aflibercept or Ranibizumab with minimal/no clinical benefit is recommended in an attempt to improve vision, reduce costs, and reduce the burden of injections of clinics and hospitals, especially in a pandemic era [16].

Author Contributions: Conceptualization, C.A., A.P.; methodology, C.A., M.G.D.; software, C.A.; validation, A.P., S.Z., F.B.; investigation, C.A., A.P.; writing—original draft preparation, C.A., M.G.D., S.D., A.P.; writing—review and editing, C.A., M.G.D., S.D., A.P.; visualization, G.B., G.C.; supervision, A.P.; funding acquisition, A.P., M.G.D. All authors have read and agreed to the published version of the manuscript.

Funding: This research received no external funding.

Institutional Review Board Statement: The study was conducted according to the guidelines of the Declaration of Helsinki. Ethical review and approval were waived for this study, due to the retrospective nature of the survey.

Informed Consent Statement: Informed consent was obtained from all subjects involved in the study.

Data Availability Statement: Data will be available upon request.

Conflicts of Interest: The authors declare no conflict of interest.

References

1. American Diabetes Association (ADA). Standards of Medical Care in Diabetes—2013. *Diabetes Care* **2013**, *36* (Suppl. 1), S11–S66. [CrossRef] [PubMed]
2. Linee Guida per lo Screening, la Diagnostica ed il Trattamento della Retinopatia Diabetica in Italia. Review and Update 2015. Available online: https://www.fondazionebietti.it/sites/default/files/pdf/lg-rd-16sett2015.pdf (accessed on 15 November 2021).
3. Acan, D.; Calan, M.; Er, D.; Arkan, T.; Kocak, N.; Bayraktar, F.; Kaynak, S. The prevalence and systemic risk factors of diabetic macular edema: A cross-sectional study from Turkey. *BMC Ophthalmol.* **2018**, *18*, 91. [CrossRef] [PubMed]
4. Virgili, G.; Menchini, F.; Murro, V.; Peluso, E.; Rosa, F.; Casazza, G. Optical coherence tomography (OCT) for detection of macular oedema in patients with diabetic retinopathy. *Cochrane Database Syst. Rev.* **2011**, *7*, CD008081.
5. Flaxel, C.J.; Adelman, R.A.; Bailey, S.T.; Fawzi, A.; Lim, J.I.; Vemulakonda, G.A.; Ying, G.-S. Diabetic Retinopathy Preferred Practice Pattern®. *Ophthalmology* **2020**, *127*, P66–P145. [CrossRef] [PubMed]
6. Klein, R.; Klein, B.E.; Moss, S.E.; Davis, M.D.; DeMets, D.L. The Wisconsin Epidemiologic Study of diabetic retinopathy III Prevalence and risk of diabetic retinopathy when age at diagnosis is 30 or more years. *Arch. Ophthalmol.* **1984**, *102*, 527–533. [CrossRef] [PubMed]
7. Klein, R.; Klein, B.E.; Moss, S.E.; Davis, M.D.; DeMets, D.L. The Wisconsin epidemiologic study of diabetic retinopathy. IX. Four-year incidence and progression of diabetic retinopathy when age at diagnosis is less than 30 years. *Arch. Ophthalmol.* **1989**, *107*, 237–243. [CrossRef] [PubMed]
8. Klein, R.; Klein, B.E.; Moss, S.E.; Cruickshanks, K.J. The Wisconsin epidemiologic study of diabetic retinopathy. X. Four-year incidence and progression of diabetic retinopathy when age at diagnosis is 30 years or more. *Arch. Ophthalmol.* **1989**, *107*, 244–249. [CrossRef] [PubMed]
9. Bhagat, N.; Grigorian, R.A.; Tutela, A.; Zarbin, M.A. Diabetic Macular Edema: Pathogenesis and Treatment. *Surv. Ophthalmol.* **2009**, *54*, 1–32. [CrossRef] [PubMed]
10. Nehmé, A.; Edelman, J. Dexamethasone inhibits high glucose-, TNF-alpha-, and IL-1beta-induced secretion of inflammatory and angiogenic mediators from retinal microvascular pericytes. *Investig. Ophthalmol. Vis. Sci.* **2008**, *49*, 2030–2038. [CrossRef] [PubMed]
11. Wang, W.; Lo, A.C.Y. Diabetic Retinopathy: Pathophysiology and Treatments. *Int. J. Mol. Sci.* **2018**, *19*, 1816. [CrossRef] [PubMed]
12. Patelli, F.; Radice, P.; Giacomotti, E. Diabetic macular edema. *Dev. Ophthalmol.* **2014**, *54*, 164–173. [PubMed]
13. Ciulla, T.A.; Amador, A.G.; Zinman, B. Diabetic Retinopathy and Diabetic Macular Edema: Pathophysiology, screening, and novel therapies. *Diabetes Care* **2003**, *26*, 2653–2664. [CrossRef] [PubMed]

14. Lee, S.S.; Hughes, P.M.; Robinson, M.R. Recent advances in drug delivery systems for treating ocular complications of systemic diseases. *Curr. Opin. Ophthalmol.* **2009**, *20*, 511–519. [CrossRef] [PubMed]
15. Boscia, F.; Giancipoli, E.; D'Amico Ricci, G.; Pinna, A. Management of macular oedema in diabetic patients undergoing cataract surgery. *Curr. Opin. Ophthalmol.* **2017**, *28*, 23–28. [CrossRef] [PubMed]
16. Iovino, C.; Peiretti, E.; Giannaccare, G.; Scorcia, V.; Carnevali, A. Evolving Treatment Paradigm in the Management of Diabetic Macular Edema in the Era of COVID-19. *Front. Pharmacol.* **2021**, *12*, 670468. [CrossRef] [PubMed]

MDPI
St. Alban-Anlage 66
4052 Basel
Switzerland
Tel. +41 61 683 77 34
Fax +41 61 302 89 18
www.mdpi.com

Journal of Clinical Medicine Editorial Office
E-mail: jcm@mdpi.com
www.mdpi.com/journal/jcm

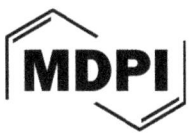

www.ingramcontent.com/pod-product-compliance
Lightning Source LLC
LaVergne TN
LVHW070554100526
838202LV00012B/460